This book is dedicated to my mom, Sandra, whose beauty evolution has always inspired me. She taught me what was important—both in beauty and in life. My favorite times with her were our "beauty nights," complete with facials, manicures and pedicures, a great old movie, and popcorn. She always told me I was beautiful—even during those awkward years. And she taught me the two most valuable life lessons: to be nice and to know that anything is possible. Thanks, Mom, for a lifetime of support.

To my mom, Sandra, whose own beauty evolution has always inspired me.

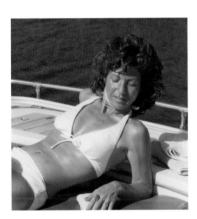
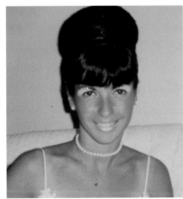
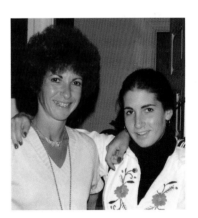
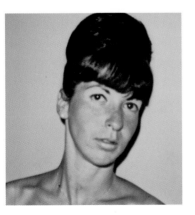
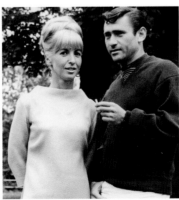
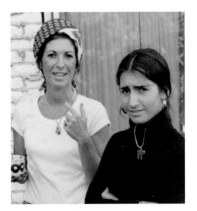

BOBBI BROWN

BOBBI BROWN

BOBBI BROWN
BEAUTY EVOLUTION

A GUIDE TO A LIFETIME OF BEAUTY
BOBBI BROWN WITH SALLY WADYKA

Aurum Press

Copyright © 2002 by Bobbi Brown Evolution LLC

First published in Great Britain
2003 by Aurum Press Ltd
25 Bedford Avenue, London WC1B 3AT

First published in 2002 by HarperCollins Publishers Inc., USA

A catalogue record for this book is available from the British Library.

ISBN 1 85410 910 3

10 9   8   7   6   5   4   3   2
2007   2006   2005   2004

Designed by Laura Shanahan
Printed and bound by Hong Kong Graphics & Printing Ltd

ACKNOWLEDGMENTS

Bobbi Brown Team

Danielle Arminio, Lisa Blair, Rochelle Bloom, Gail Boyé, Candice Burd, Joe Caracappa, Maureen Case, Tiffany Cavallaro, Tracy Davis, Danielle Dineen, Tara Eisenberg, Hazel Elardo, Mimi Field, Megan Fletcher, Margaux Guérard, Maria Keerd, Hollie Levy, Jessica Liebeskind, Erica Lyons, Dorothy Mancuso, Judith Maxfield, Beryl Meyer, Gabrielle Nevin, Curtis Phelps, Jessica Rosenbloom, Ellice Schwab, Bill Shaffer, Marie Clare Sillick, Barbara Stone, Sebastien Tardif, Alexis Varbero, Jillian Veran, Ralph Vestbom, Cynde Watson.

Other thanks

Julie Adams, A. Smaltz Inc. Modeling Agency, Nidhi Adhiya, Aida Angjeli, Anne Klein (Sue Furboter), Kathy Aruzzo, Emily Baker, Martha Baker, Banana Republic (Michelle Hellman and Kim Sobel), Bryan Bantry Modeling Agency, Lucia Bedarida Servadio, Deborah H. Berkowitz, Carmen Berra, Yogi Berra, Bitten, Angelica Bocour, Nicola Bocour, Nina Bocour, Lorraine Bracco, Joanne Bronander, James Brown, Lola Brown, John Cali, Rose Cali, Susana Canario, CarolLee Carruth, Mary Randolph Carter, Donna Cerutto, Alva Chinn, Nancy M. Clayman, Click Modeling Agency, Clotilde, Krista Cohen, Susan Cole, Gina Coleman, Carmen Dell'Orefice, Dianne DeWitt, DNA modeling agency, Dr. Jeanine B. Downie, Jeane S. Eddy, Nicole Eisenberg, Elite Modeling Agency, Lauren Ezersky, Bernice Feldman, Angie Feliciano, Han Feng, Frances B. Ferlauto, Claudia Ferrera, Angelique Flynn, Anne Fontaine-Patrice Keitt, Ford Modeling Agency, Dr. Bryan Forley, Susan Forristal, Allison Gandolfo, The Gap (Jen Listelat), Marilyn Gaultier Modeling Agency, Giorgio Armani Collezione, Jean Godfrey-June, Johanna Greenfield, Deirdre Guest, Lisa Hahnebach-Nevins, Betty Halbreich, Jeanette Hallen, Kym Hampton, Mona S. Hanley, Bethann Hardison, Christina Harvey, Mica Hatsushima, Mariann Higgins, Ronald Hill, Susan Hill, Grethe B. Holby, Alex Huang, ID Modeling Agency, IMG Modeling Agency, Industria Studios, Rosemary Iversen, Julie Jackson, Aisha Jafar, Lee Ann Jefferies, Cindy Joseph, Julia Joseph, Nanjoo Joung, Stacey S. Joyce, Ranjana Khan, Miriam Katigbak, Judy Kaufman, Stella Keitel, Lisa Knowlton, Harry Kong, Sylvia Krechevsky, Norma Borja Kroll, Jackie Kwon, Leslie Larson, Amy Lazarus, Betsy Lembeck, Wendy Lewis, Shirley Lord, Barbara Lubar, Colleen Lyons, Kathleen Macneill-Abruzzo, Madison Modeling Agency, Brian Magallones, Lee Heh Margolies, Deirdre Maguire, Lorraine

Mattheus, Judith McGhee, Susan McGraw, Liraz Mesilaty, Felicia Milewicz, Marek Milewicz, Sharron Miller, Christopher Morris, Mary Muggli, Denise Muggli, Cindy Muggli, Ilona Murane, Next Modeling Agency, Greta Nikiteas, Chandra North, *O Magazine*, Scott Ohsay, Javier Ortega, Ruth Perretti, Ruth D. Perretti, Bonnie Pfeifer, Dickie Plofker, Morton & Evelyn Plofker, Steven Plofker, Richard Plofker, Sandra Woodward Pullman, Q Modeling Agency, Sabrina Randall, Nikki Ray, Marisabel R. Raymond, Sandra Redrick, Erica H. Reid, Jamie Rivera, Deborah Roberts, Leah Robins, Aandre Rodman, Susanna Romano, Amy M. Rosen, Selma Rosen, Mary Beth Rosenthal, Yasmine Rossi, Colleen Kaehr Saidman, Gabriella Sanchez, Paola Saunders, Pamela Scott, Tara Segall, Anna Maria Shanahan, Anna Shillinglaw, Ruth Sigua, Audrey Smaltz, Susan G. Smith, Soho Studios, Michelle Stevens, Jean Strahan, Michael Strahan, Theresa Swabson, Cynthia Swabsin, Takashi, Dara Torres, Dorothea Towles, TSE Cashmere (Terence Charles), Mia Tyler, Justine Van der Leun, Priya Virmani, Pamela Wakefield, Saskia Webber, Heidi Weisel, Eileen Weller, Kim Whittam, Wilhelmina New York Modeling Agency, Women Modeling Agency, Yogi Berra Museum.

Special Acknowledgments
Sally Wadyka for getting my words just so.
Tara Eisenberg for doing everything effortlessly.
Cathy Lempert and Betty Ann Grund for finding such great women.
Laura Shanahan for sharing my vision.
Patricia Van der Leun for her guidance and believing in me.
Kathy Huck and Megan Newman for their enthusiasm and direction.
Lise Varrette for her special portraits.
Ernesto Urdaneta for his awesome beauty shots.
Rick Burda for his beautiful stills and great candids.
Jean-Bernard Villareal for his great behind-the-scenes shots.
Especially Walter Chin for his friendship and stunning photos.

And to my family, Steven, Dylan, Dakota, and Duke, who put up with me and love and support me. And always, my dad, James Brown, who knows how much I love him.

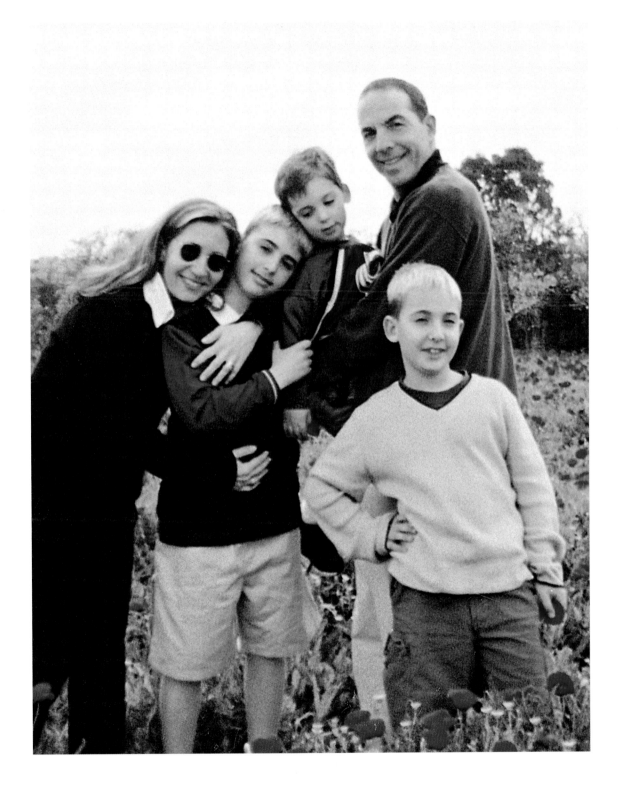

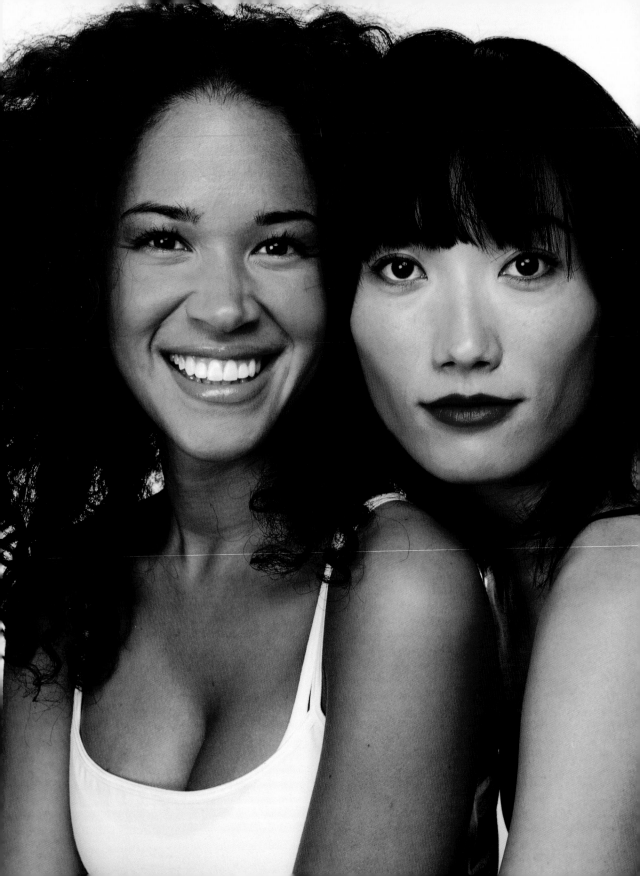

CONTENTS

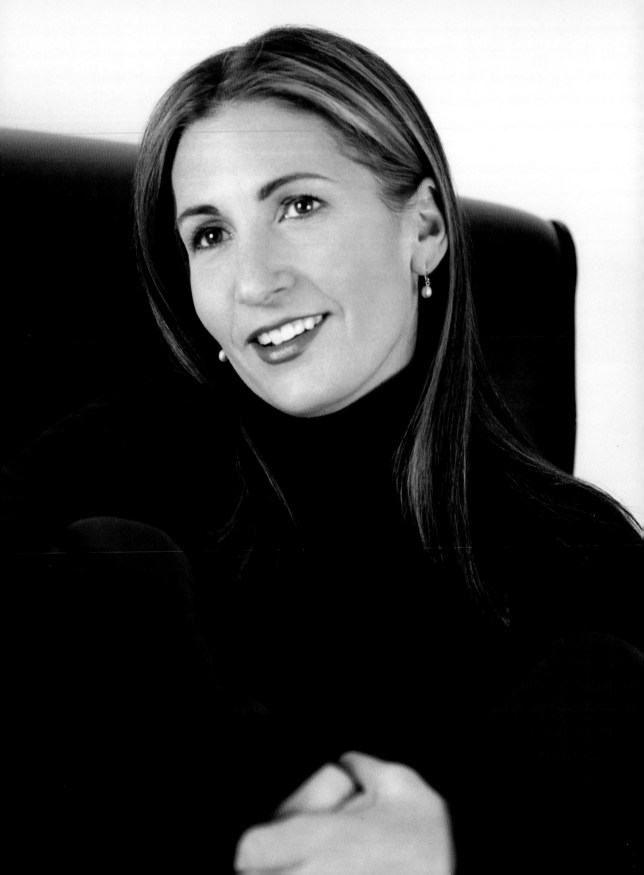

BOBBI'S OWN EVOLUTION

This book is about our constant evolution and the changes that come with each passing year. It's about what happens as we make our way through life and how we can continue making ourselves better. Women—whether they're models, actresses, CEOs, friends, moms, grandmothers, or aunts—all crave the same thing: to look pretty and feel good. I know because I spend my life with women and listen to their complaints, their desires, and their dreams.

As I sit down to write this book, I am right in the middle of my forties. But sometimes I still feel like I'm not quite an adult. I still respect my elders. I still wear my long-sleeve sweaters so that they almost entirely cover my hands. (And I still hear my mother saying not to.) I still want my dad's approval. I still want to be liked. I still want to be five pounds lighter (and four inches taller!). But here I am, a "grown-up." I am happily married, have three great kids, a home, and a successful business.

Sometimes I look in the mirror or at photographs of myself and say, "You look good, girl." And I sometimes look at photos or tapes of TV appearances and say, "Yikes!" But at forty-five, I honestly only feel thirty, and I am quite surprised when I look in the mirror and don't see myself at thirty. I'm not saying that I love the fine lines I see on my face or catching a glimpse of my profile (which I've never liked too much). I still think my chest is too big for my body, and I've never loved my arms. But the good news is that I've reached a point in my life where I feel like it's all okay. I am who I am. I'm comfortable with my style—classic silhouettes, simple jewelry, glowing makeup. And most importantly, I am comfortable in my own skin. And that, I think, is my secret, as well as the secret of many happy people I know.

I've reached a point in my life where I feel like it's all okay. I am who I am.

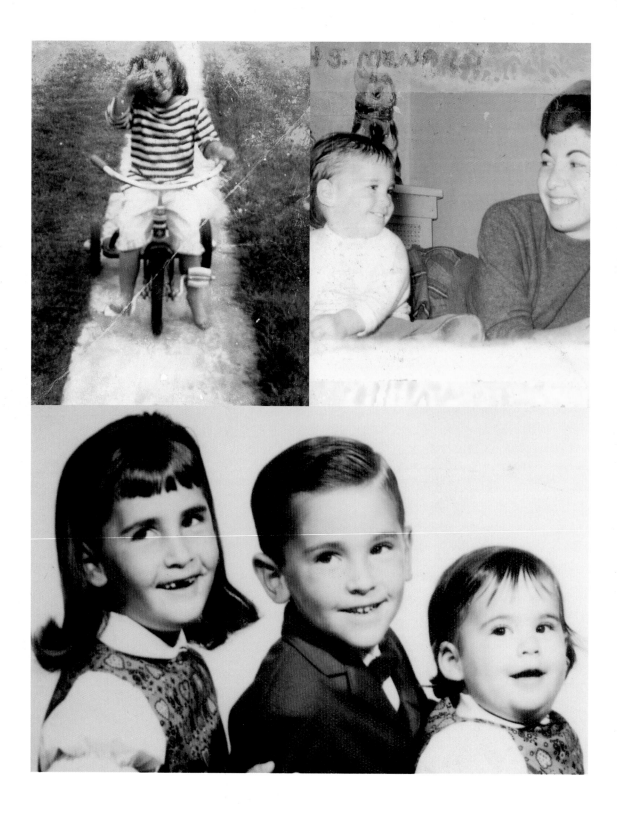

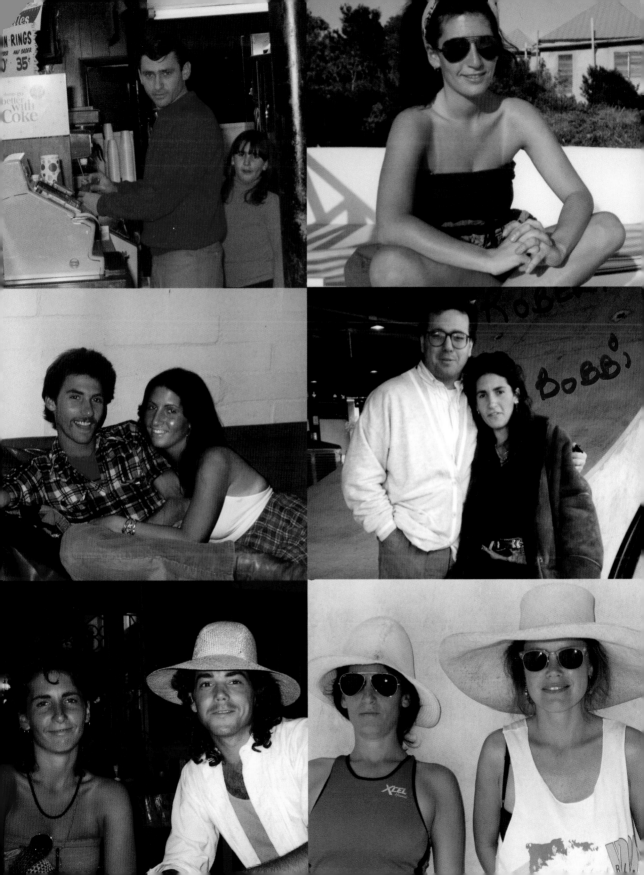

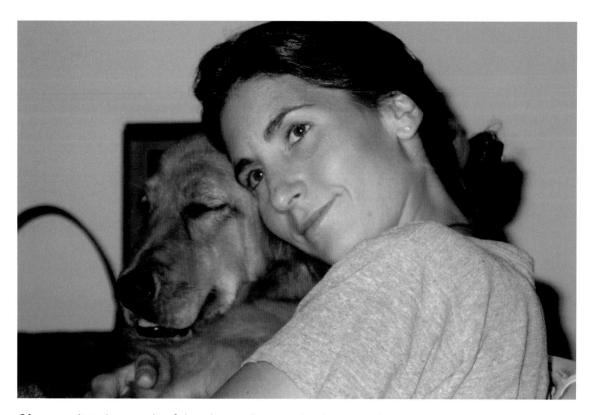

Of course, it took a couple of decades—and many mistakes—to get where I am today. Coming to New York in my twenties as a young makeup artist, I worked all day surrounded by models and mirrors. That was hard. No matter how good I thought I looked when I left the house in the morning, I'd get to the studio and feel like I didn't have it together. Every day I experimented with my clothes and hair and makeup, trying to figure out who I was and how I wanted to look. My turning point came at age thirty-two, when I was pregnant with my first child and feeling really lumpy. I was working at a bathing suit fashion show. I looked up and saw Christy Turlington, Linda Evangelista, and Cindy Crawford in bikinis. I said to myself, "Don't go there!" I made a decision that I couldn't for a second feel bad about myself because of the way *they* looked.

Over the years, I've learned to go with the flow. Whether I'm in an important business meeting, backstage at a fashion show, on TV, or even at an Oscar party, the trick is to take a deep breath, do your best, and just be yourself. I realized years ago that I couldn't compete in the looks department with models, actresses, or those near-perfect friends. But I can put all I've learned together to make myself feel and look better. And the purpose of this book is to share my tips and help all women begin to appreciate who they are.

My philosophy is that all women have the ability to be their best. That's why I chose to photograph so many women (mostly non-models) of all shapes, sizes, and ages for this book. Looking your best is a combination of acquiring knowledge (some great tricks and techniques), accepting the things you can't change, and having confidence in yourself. It's a matter of learning to enjoy your life and feeling good about who you are.

I want every woman who reads this book to put it down feeling better about herself. So much of what we see in the media makes us feel bad about ourselves—because we don't have the perfect body, skin, hair, or whatever. Of course, there are plenty of things you can do to make yourself feel and look better (just read the rest of the book and you'll learn them all!), but first you need self-confidence. Beauty is the result of realizing what is special about you and not focusing on the things you don't like.

The good news: Looking your best is so simple and so achievable. It takes an open mind, some good advice, and a little work, but you can do it! XXO

Bobbi

Beauty is the result of realizing what is special about you.

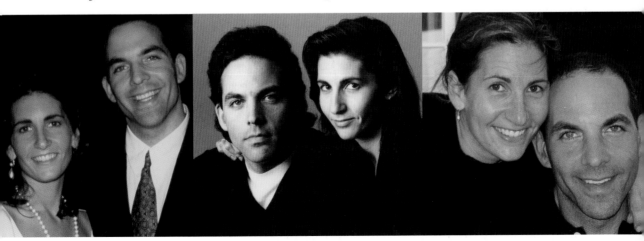

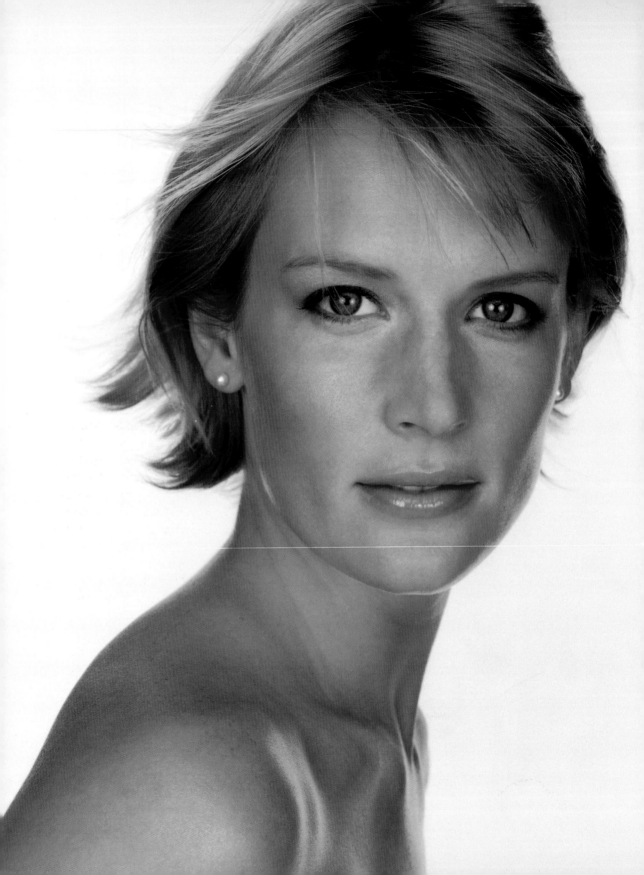

1 BEAUTY ILLUSION VS. BEAUTY REALITY

You are probably aware of this already, but it's worth repeating: What you see in magazines doesn't always portray reality. A whole team of makeup artists, hairstylists, fashion stylists, photographers, art directors (and later, photo retouchers) work hard to create a beautiful illusion. Yes, it's pretty to look at. But is it real? Absolutely not. I'm not suggesting that the models and celebrities you see in magazines aren't beautiful. Of course they are, but they're also human. And just like you and me, they often have dark circles under their eyes, uneven patches on their skin, blemishes, hair where it's not supposed to be, or other imperfections. By the time all the experts get through with them, the result is an image of perfection. But most of them do not walk into a photo session looking that way.

This is especially important to remember as you get older and look at images of older women. The media doesn't seem to like letting women show their age. So even those who haven't had their faces surgically retouched often end up having them digitally retouched. So be careful when you look at a photograph of a model or actress who is your age but magically has none of the lines on her face that you have. Keep in mind that a lot of people went to a lot of trouble to ensure you don't see those lines!

The photograph below demonstrates retouching in process. The photo at left shows the finished product.

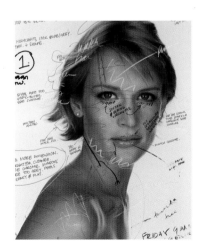

Behind the Scenes with the Magicians of the Photo Shoot
Let the industry insiders tell you what really goes into the "perfect" images they produce.

Bobbi Brown
"Makeup at a photo shoot is very different from makeup you would wear out on the street. Even though I use the same cosmetics for both situations, they are used very differently. The way I apply foundation depends on the lighting of the shoot. Inside a photography studio where the lighting is very strong, the foundation has to be dense to create an extreme version of flawless skin. For close-up beauty shots, I apply a ton of concealer, foundation, and powder to cover everything. It looks great in a photo, but in real life it would

look too fake. In order for natural-looking shades to show up at all in a photo, they have to be applied with a heavy hand and then blended really well. Eyes, lips, and cheeks have to be colored stronger than you'd ever wear otherwise. And one of the makeup tricks used for photography that never works in real life is contouring. I will use dark shades to create the illusion of a different-shaped nose, sculpted cheekbones, or a thinner chin. If anyone tried to walk outside like that, she'd look like she had smudges of dirt on her face."

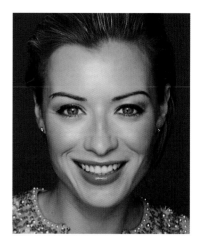

Felicia Milewicz, Beauty Director, *Glamour*

"At a photo shoot, amazing miracles are created. So few models come to the shoot with great complexions, but the makeup artist can create a perfect, flawless canvas out of the face. The makeup artist is like the plastic surgeon of the set. And the makeup and the lighting together are what create the illusion you see in the photograph. Even with that, nearly every photo that ends up in a magazine is retouched to some degree. I think retouching is very tragic because, in a way, they are removing people's personalities. They're removing their lives from their faces because lines are like a road map of our lives. We've earned whatever's there—the happiness, sadness, ups and downs. And maybe it's not beautiful in the way we normally think of the word, but it is beautiful because it is real and it represents our emotions."

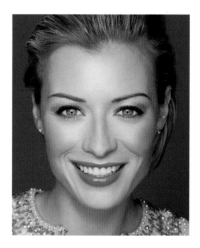

These photos illustrate the miracle of retouching.

Clotilde, Model

"The most important thing to realize is that when an expert photographer lights a set, he can create a wonderful illusion. You could put anyone under those lights and they're going to look gorgeous. And then of course, there's the retouching. Sometimes I would do a shoot for a beauty ad and later open up the magazine, see the photo, and think that's not me! You can't even believe how good it looks. Photos like that are almost like making an illustration."

Walter Chin, Photographer

"To me, a striking and interesting face, not one that is flawless or pretty, is the key component to creating a beautiful photo. Makeup, hair, lighting, which I use as a sculpting tool for enhancement, are important in helping to create the beauty in the final print. But most importantly, I have to find the innate beauty in who I am photographing; without that insight, I will fail to achieve a portrait of what I consider true beauty."

Jon Rosen, Photo Retoucher

"The looks now being achieved in photographs could never be achieved in real life. It's above and beyond cosmetic clean-up. It's taken for granted that you will get rid of lines and eye bags. There's a hyper-realism in photography now that demands more post-production work. One thing that is commonly done is that faces are reassembled from various parts—taking the eyes you like from one shot and the smile from another and putting them together to create a perfect face. It's an exaggerated perfection, and something that no human being could ever look like."

Laura Shanahan, Art Director

"When I was a teenager, I used to read fashion magazines cover to cover, wondering how all the models could possibly be so perfect. Now I know the secret: good lighting and retouching! Don't get me wrong—models are beautiful and have lovely hair and skin. It's just that they deal with the same issues we mortals do—blemishes, dark circles, etc. Film tends to enhance it all. Whenever I am working with a photo of a model, I automatically have the retoucher do a general clean-up on the photo, whitening the eyes and teeth, zapping any blemishes and facial hair, and smoothing under eye circles. The results are amazing, as you can see here."

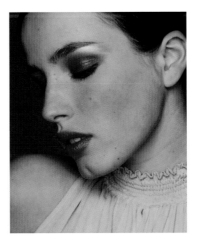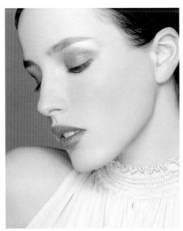

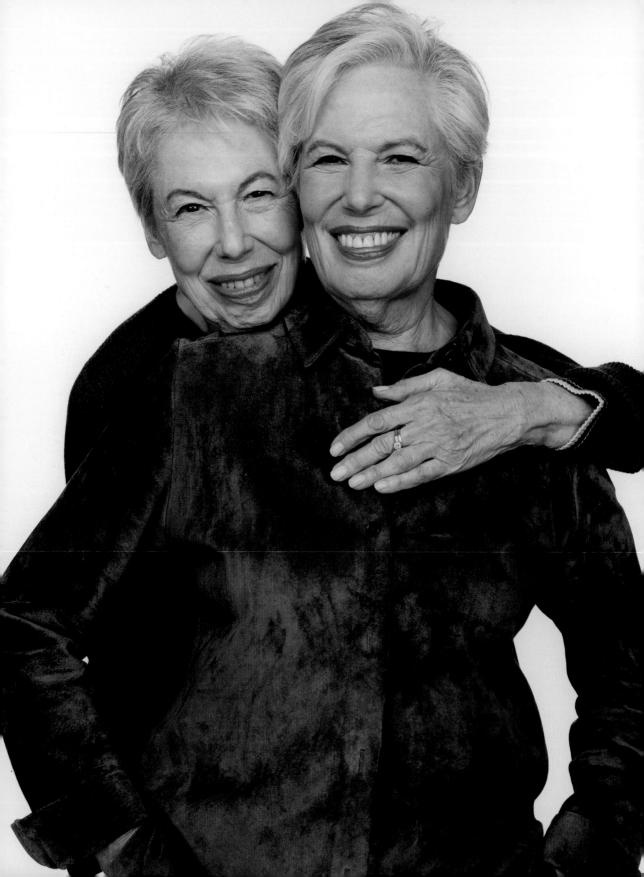

2 BEAUTY ODYSSEY:
TWO SISTERS SHARE THEIR PHOTO ALBUM

Bernice (a.k.a. Bunny) Feldman, who's seventy-eight years old, and her little sister Selma Rosen, seventy-two, have been best friends their entire lives. They've grown up together, traveled together, and celebrated together for more than seven decades. A glimpse into their photo album reveals what a beautiful journey it has been (and continues to be).

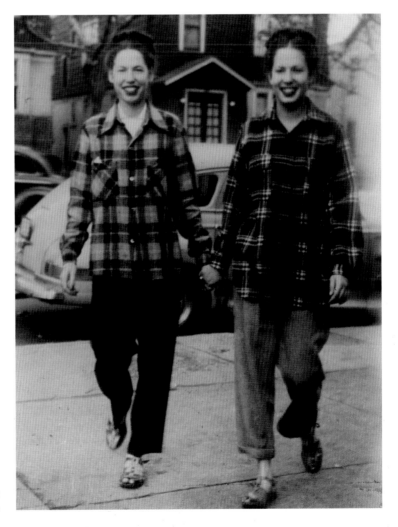

Bernice and Selma today (left) and in 1945 (right).

Bunny's and Selma's Thoughts on Beauty

When did you feel the most beautiful?
Selma: "When my first child was born."

What's the best thing about being the age you are now?
Selma: "You don't have to try to look like you're twenty."
Bunny: "I get to share my life with my children and my grandchildren."

What are the beauty problems that come with your age?
Selma: "Bags under my eyes and wrinkles around my mouth."
Bunny: "Droopy eyes and triple chins."

What makes you feel beautiful?
Selma: "Being with my husband."

What gives you confidence?
Bunny: "Looking good and being surrounded by friends and family."

Who do you think is truly beautiful?
Selma: "My children and grandchildren because they are so alive and involved and loving."
Bunny: "My sister, Selma, because she is a good and caring person."

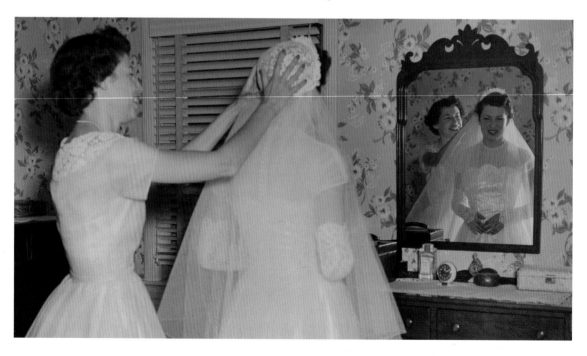

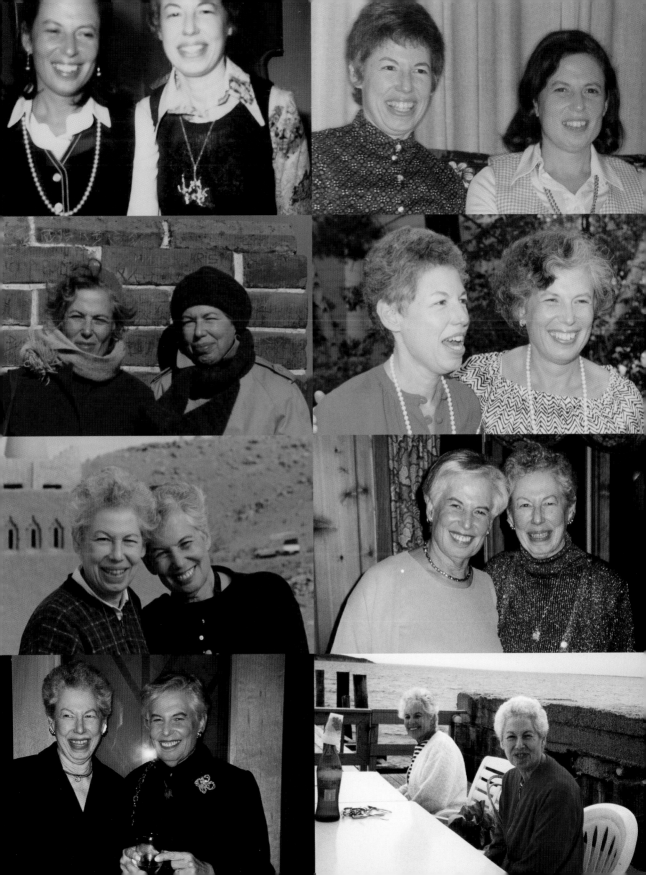

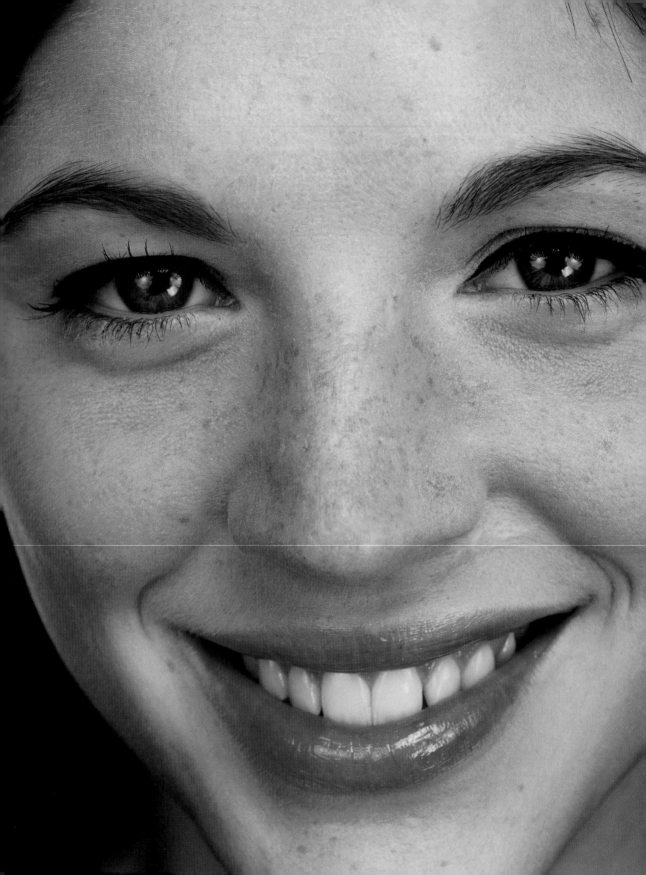

3 YOUR TWENTIES

The twenties is a physically beautiful decade (it's no coincidence that most models are in their twenties). But the one thing too many women in their twenties are missing—no matter how beautiful they are—is self-confidence. I promise that you will one day look back to your twenties and say, "I shouldn't have been so critical of myself. I really looked good!" The most important advice I can give you is to look in the mirror and try to appreciate what you see. Self-confidence is what makes a woman look truly attractive (and what guarantees that no one else notices your so-called flaws like a blemish or an extra five pounds). It is difficult to achieve that kind of self-awareness at this age because, for most women, their twenties is a time of tremendous change and uncertainty. Even if you don't have a lot of insecurities about your looks, you may have insecurities about where you are in your life and how you will get to where you want to be. This is the decade when you make the transition from student to grown-up, when you stop being a girl and become a woman, when you start working on your career and possibly get married.

This is the decade when you make the transition from student to grown-up.

Part of this transition is finding your own style, an image you feel comfortable with. And the twenties is the decade you spend trying to do that—experimenting with different hairstyles, trying every fashion trend, and wearing crazy makeup colors. This is the time to have fun with all that, but it's also time to start thinking about who you are and how you want to look. Some of this may be dictated by your career choice: Acceptable looks differ in different professional environments, so it's not a bad idea to take a cue from the women you work with. My early role models were stylists and women in the fashion industry, like Mary Randolph Carter and Ricky Lauren. I tried to emulate their classic, pretty, minimalist look and quickly realized this was how I felt most comfortable. This may be the first time you start to realize the way you look is an important factor when it comes to getting you where you want to go in life. I'm not saying it's a good thing, but it's the truth: People do judge you on the way you look.

And for your career, that means presenting an image that fits your chosen field. In other words, the super-trendy clothes and makeup that may look right for a fashion magazine job are all wrong at a law firm. (See chapter 23 for interview-appropriate makeup advice.)

What You Need to Know Now

This is the time to start getting serious about skin care. You should be learning good habits that'll help your skin your whole life, such as always wearing sunscreen, never going to bed with your makeup on, and using the right cleansing products for your skin type. In general, the twenties is when the focus of skin care should be on cleansing and prevention. You need to keep skin clean and pores unclogged in order to help avoid breakouts. Cleansers that contain salicylic or glycolic acid are a good bet because they help skin exfoliate, clearing dead cells from pores on a daily basis. But be wary of overdrying your skin, a common mistake made by young blemish-prone women. When you attempt to zap every bit of oil away, your glands respond by pumping out even more. The result: dry, flaky skin that's still greasy and breaking out. If skin does feel dry, moisturize with an oil-free lotion that won't clog pores. (See chapter 13 for more skin care tips.)

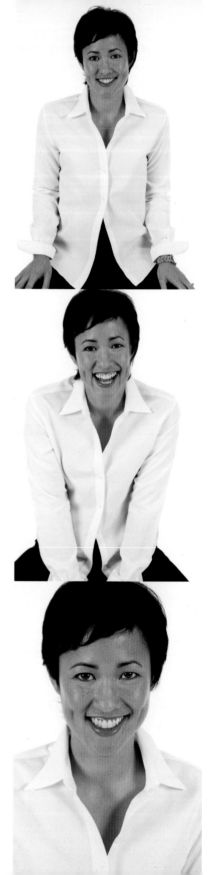

This is also a good time to become diligent with sunscreen. Chances are, whatever sun damage you've accumulated so far hasn't shown up on your face yet, but unfortunately, it will by the time you hit your mid-thirties. To avoid any more damage, start wearing sunscreen—at least SPF 15—every day, rain or shine, winter or summer. At the beach, protect your face with a baseball cap in addition to sunscreen of SPF 30 or more. Believe me, ten years from now, when your skin is still unlined and unfreckled, you'll be glad you did!

You should also start investing in a few key makeup items. Foundation and concealer are the two biggies, and those are the items you really should spend money on. Lipstick, nail polish, even eye shadow can be bought at the drugstore, but I don't think you can get a good foundation or concealer for a few dollars. You might buy the perfect foundation for $30, or three bad ones for $12 apiece, so it's actually cheaper to invest in the one that's right for your skin. Plus, if you find the right one, it will last you at least a year. (See chapter 16 for tips on picking out and applying foundation and concealer.)

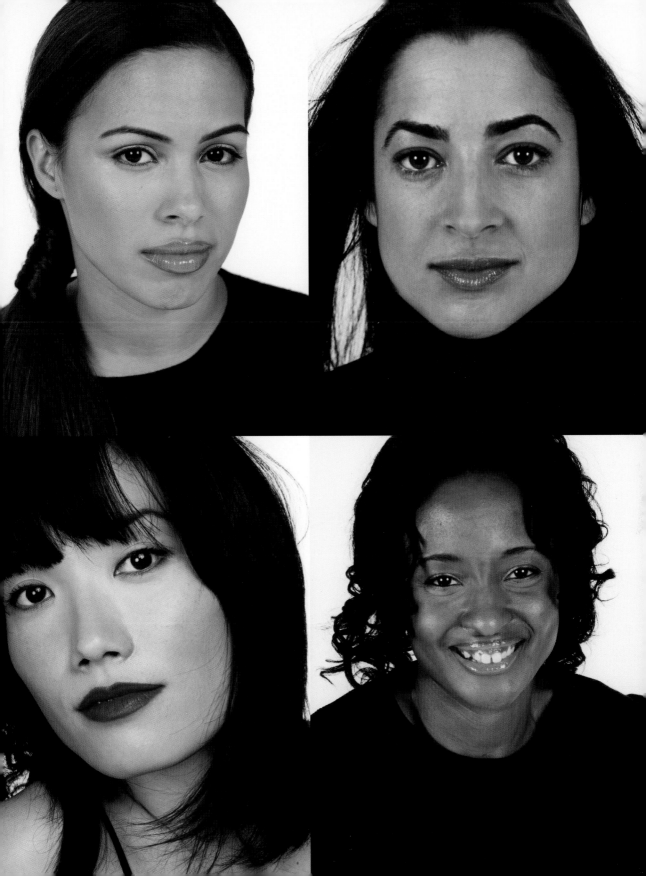

Bobbi's Essentials for Your Twenties

- **Sunscreen:** Save your skin now! The sun damage you do in your twenties will show up in your thirties, forties, and beyond.
- **A good cleanser:** If drugstore brands aren't keeping your skin clear, see a dermatologist to get a more potent product.
- **Eye cream:** The skin around your eyes shows signs of aging first, so keep it well hydrated and protected.
- **Concealer:** A must-have for disguising under-eye circles the morning after a too-late night.
- **Tinted moisturizer:** Lighter than foundation, it'll smooth out skin tone and give skin a nice glow.
- **Stick foundation:** This is the best way to cover blemishes. Just make sure the shade is an exact match for your skin, or you will end up drawing more attention to the spot you are trying to hide. (See chapter 16 for a step-by-step technique to disguise blemishes.)

"THE BEST THING ABOUT BEING THIS AGE IS THAT I AM BECOMING A WOMAN BUT AM STILL ABLE TO GET AWAY WITH BEING A GIRL." —JULIA, AGE 27

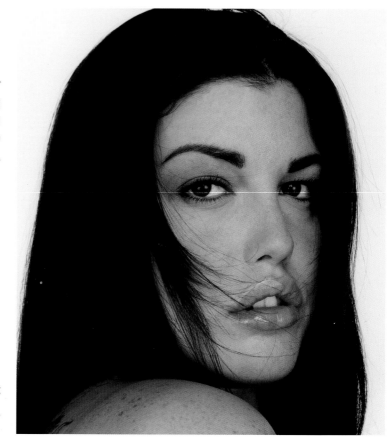

Model and actress Mia Tyler looking beautifully natural, right, and with a more dramatic, rock-'n'-roll-worthy smoky eye, far right.

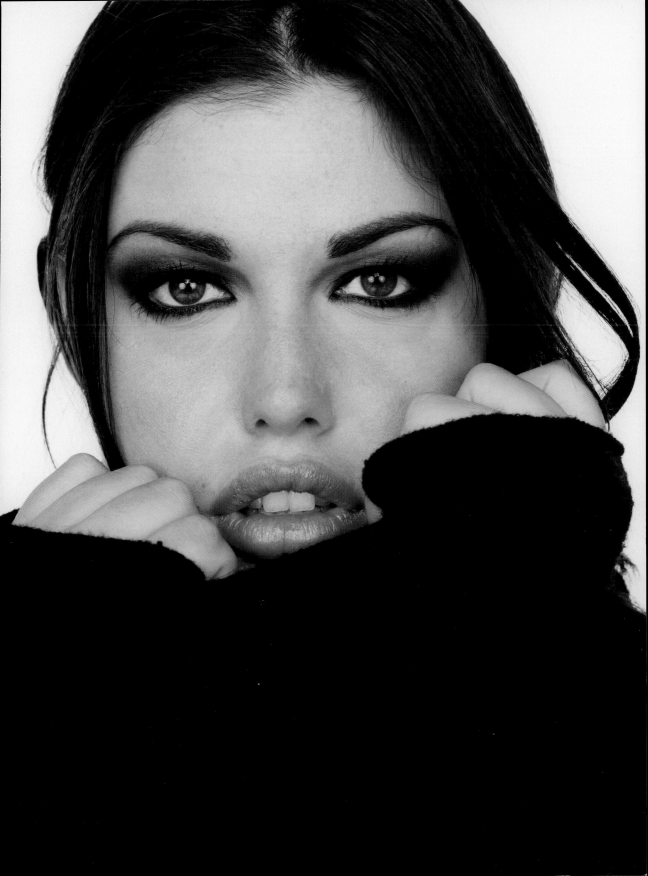

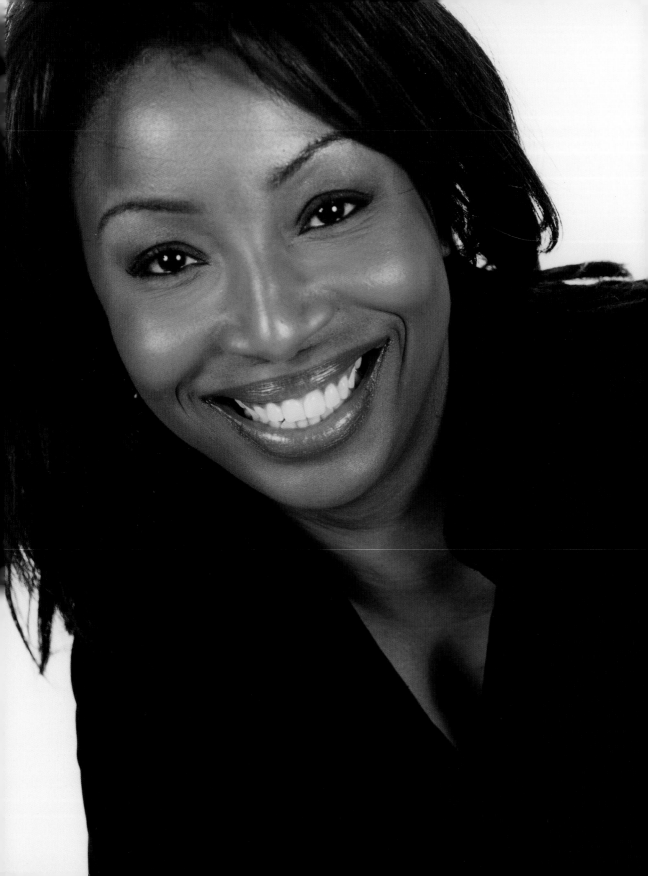

4 YOUR THIRTIES

This is the great multitasking decade. Career, home, family—you're trying to have it all. That is why this is often a decade of feeling overwhelmed: Working women with kids worry they aren't giving enough time to either their career or their family; women who are postponing having children to focus on their careers stress out because they think they should be concentrating on starting a family; and everyone worries about pushing themselves harder to look better and do more. It's usually in your early thirties that you first have the shocking realization that all the bad stuff you did in your twenties—staying out late, not exercising, frying in the sun—really does have an impact. You might see the first tiny lines on your face or freckly spots on your skin, and maybe your metabolism starts to slow down a bit. Relax. It's a normal part of getting older and is not the end of the world (not to mention there's still plenty of time to get back on the right track to taking better care of yourself).

Now is definitely not the time to get obsessive about your little flaws. In your thirties, you should be more proactive about taking care of yourself than you were in your twenties—eat well, exercise regularly, and protect your skin—but it's also a time to let go of some of the things that used to seem important. I remember when I was in my twenties I was very concerned about where my tan lines were, and that's the kind of obsession you should definitely outgrow when you hit your thirties. You've probably made most of your style mistakes already, and now you're ready to spend a bit more money on the makeup you know will work, a good haircut, and the right hair color.

What You Need to Know Now
If you didn't get into the sunscreen habit in your twenties, you really need to step up your vigilance now. In order to prevent lines and minimize sun damage and skin aging, you need to wear an SPF of 15 or 30 on your face every day. Find a moisturizer that has a sunscreen built in or wear it underneath your moisturizer, but wear it! It's the single best thing you can do for your skin. You might want to see a dermatologist to find out about products and treatments that can help minimize fine lines and freshen your skin, such as Retin-A and glycolic acid peels. (See chapter 13 for skin care tips and chapter 25 for line-softening tricks.) Hormonal fluctuations may cause occa-

sional breakouts (especially right before your period), so you will need to contend with fighting blemishes and wrinkles simultaneously. To avoid overdrying your skin in an effort to prevent breakouts, use oil-free moisturizers and gentle acne products made for adult skin (ones with salicylic acid are a good bet).

You need to wear an SPF of 15 or 30 every day.

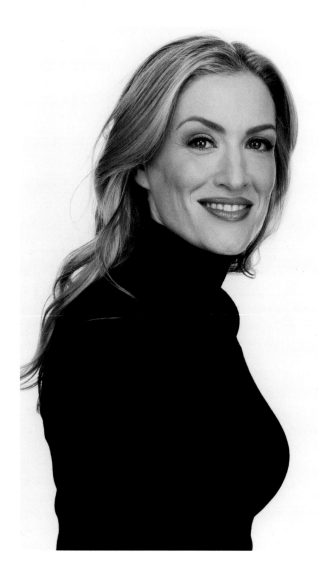

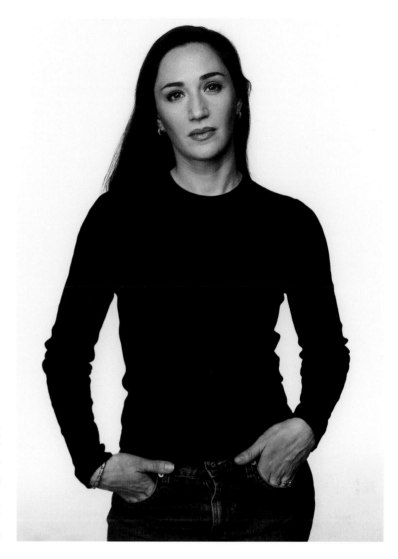

"I'M MORE
CONFIDENT AND HAPPY
WITH MYSELF AS I GET
OLDER. SO I LOVE IT
WHEN PEOPLE ASK
ME MY AGE."
—ELLICE, AGE 36 (RIGHT)

As for makeup, products that do double duty (like tinted moisturizer) or that are quick to use (like eyebrow groomer or lipstick you can apply without looking in the mirror) can be lifesavers during these hectic years. You want things that make you look put together in an instant because whether you're juggling three kids or working twelve hours a day, what most women in their thirties have in common is a lack of time for themselves. One of my favorite tricks is taking a makeup palette and filling it with a few essentials—stick foundation, cream blush, lip balm, and one or two lip colors. That way you can have all you really need to look polished right in the palm of your hand.

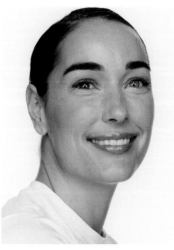

- **A good moisturizer (with SPF 15 or higher):** Use it every day. If skin is still oily or blemish-prone, choose one that's oil-free.
- **Eye cream:** The area around your eyes will start getting noticeably drier, so using eye cream before applying concealer is essential.
- **Concealer**
- **Foundation**
- **Two blushes:** Use one that blends effortlessly into skin, another that's a shade brighter to wake up your face (see chapter 18 for tips on picking the right shades).
- **A neutral lip color:** Choose a shade you can put on without looking.
- **A cosmetic bag filled with essentials:** Keep it in your purse, so you're always ready to go.
- **Face-cleansing wipes:** Use these for removing makeup in a hurry when you don't even have time to wash your face.

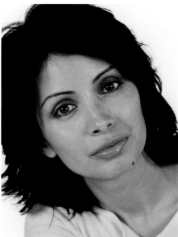

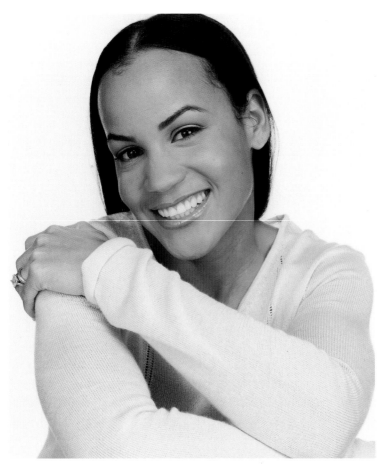

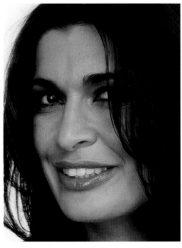

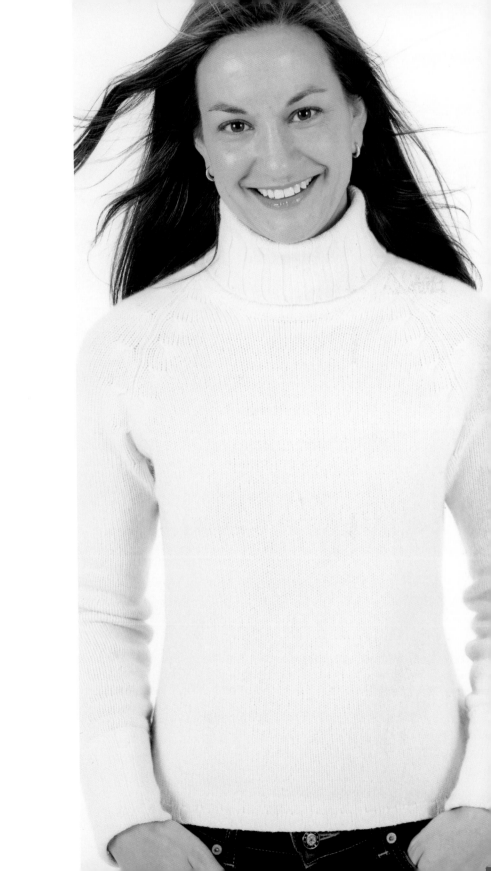

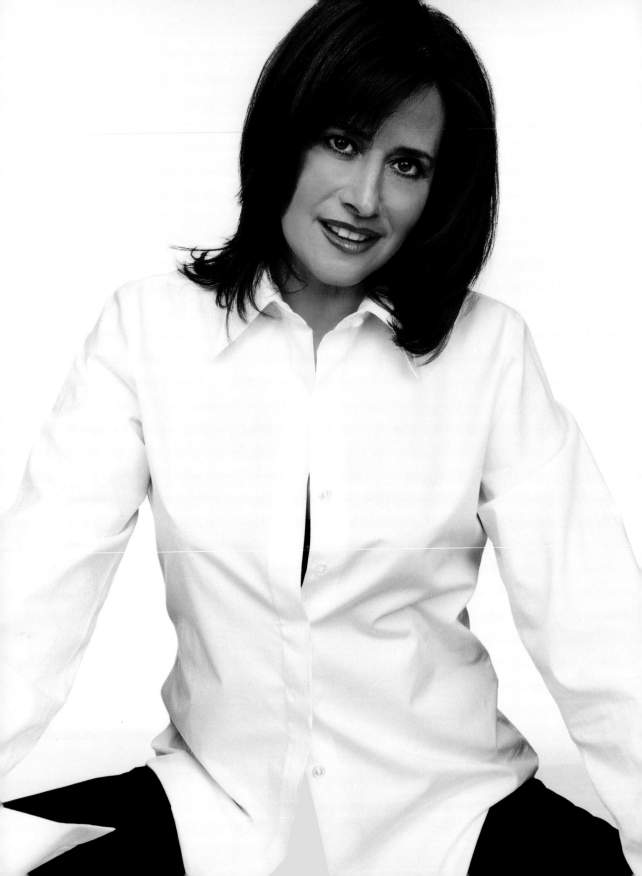

5 YOUR FORTIES

This is where I am now—smack in the middle of my forties. If I had to sum up the decade so far, I'd say this is definitely the "oh shit decade." It's when you first notice that you actually do look older than you used to. But the good news is that now I am better able to appreciate when I look good, and I'm less critical and a lot more realistic than I used to be. Your forties is when you finally start coming to terms with things you can't change—and figure out how to improve the things you can, by wearing the right styles, doing your makeup and hair a certain way, and finding what makes you feel confident. I wish I'd felt this way in my thirties, but better late than never!

Your forties is not the time for being trendy. It's about being classic—in clothes and makeup—but not boring. You can still take the trends and make them wearable. For example, if the trend is fuchsia lips, then try a brighter berry lipstick. And in fashion, you can follow trends, but not to the extreme. You want to look like a chic forty-year-old, not like you're trying to be eighteen again. Hopefully you have figured out your style and are able to buy less, but buy better.

You'll have to spend a bit more time on yourself when you get to your forties. It's harder to just roll out of bed and look good. You don't have to have an elaborate hairstyle and full makeup all the time, but a little something can go a long way. I can still get away with no makeup if my hair is done nicely; or I can go out with wet hair pulled back in a ponytail, but only if I've got a little concealer, blush, and lipstick on. There are tricks you can start using in your forties to make yourself look fresher. It's not about looking younger (although, certainly, some things can make you look younger); it's about looking fresher, prettier, better. Covering your gray with a few highlights around your face can do wonders, and even just getting a hair gloss for extra shine gives your looks a boost. But most essential is a good cut. Invest in one and take the time to learn how to style it—even if that means purchasing a few new styling products or tools because the right products and brushes can make all the difference in how your hair looks.

What You Need to Know Now

The right moisturizer becomes crucial during this decade (and beyond). A lot of women start getting dry skin in their forties; it's the time when even oily skin becomes a little dehydrated. You should switch to a heavier cream. A good trick for days when you feel extra dry is taking a bit of dense cream, rubbing it between your palms, and then patting it onto your skin after you've done your makeup. It adds that fresh, dewy look you used to have naturally when you were younger. Depending on your skin, you might also feel like you need to start wearing more makeup. I always hesitate to tell people "more" because it's really about wearing the right makeup, not more of products that aren't working to begin with. You will definitely start to see more red tones in your skin than you did in your twenties or thirties, so a good foundation becomes worth its weight in gold. The trick is to find a yellow-toned foundation that evens out your skin, disguises redness, and still looks completely natural. (See chapter 16 for foundation basics.) This is the decade when you may begin to notice that your face looks a bit washed out. It's amazing what the right blush can do. (See chapter 18 for help with choosing colors.) A little more definition on your eyes will perk up your look, too. It doesn't have to be strong color; even just mascara or a simple brown eyeliner can make a big difference.

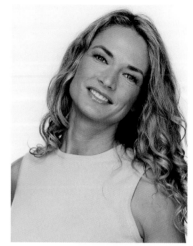

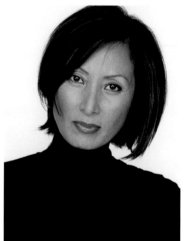

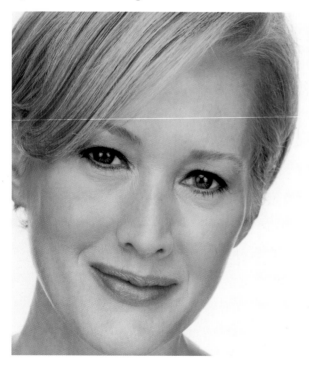

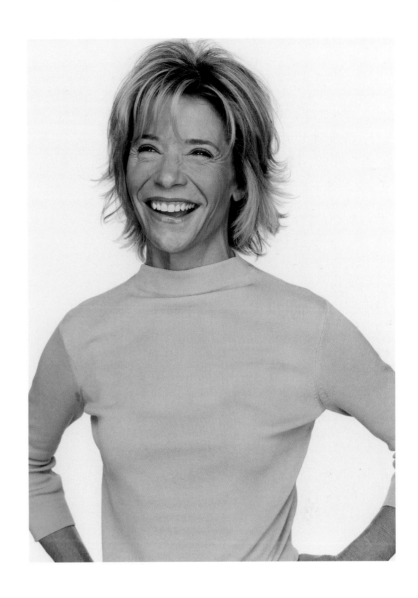

"I AM SELF-CONSCIOUS OF MY CROOKED SMILE, MY DROOPY EYELID, THE SCARS ON MY NECK. THEY ARE ALL THE RESULT OF BEING BRUTALLY ATTACKED WHEN I WAS TWENTY. MOSTLY I'M JUST GLAD TO HAVE SURVIVED, BUT BECAUSE OF THAT EXPERIENCE, I DON'T REALLY TRUST OUTER BEAUTY. I FEEL BEAUTIFUL WHEN I'M LAUGHING, WHEN I MAKE OTHER PEOPLE HAPPY, AND WHEN I'M SMART ENOUGH TO REALIZE HOW LUCKY I AM." —LEAH, AGE 45 (ABOVE)

Bobbi's Essentials for Your Forties

- **SPF lotion:** It's not too late to prevent additional sun damage.
- **Eye cream:** It's a must to make your concealer go on smoothly.
- **Moisturizer:** You may need to switch to a slightly heavier formula (although if skin still breaks out, keep it oil-free).
- **Concealer:** It wakes up tired eyes.
- **Foundation:** It can cover redness and even out skin tone.
- **Blush:** Your skin may no longer have a natural glow, so add it back.
- **Eye liner and mascara:** It can add definition to eyes.
- **Hair color:** It can brighten your face, whether you add just a few highlights or do all-over color to cover gray.

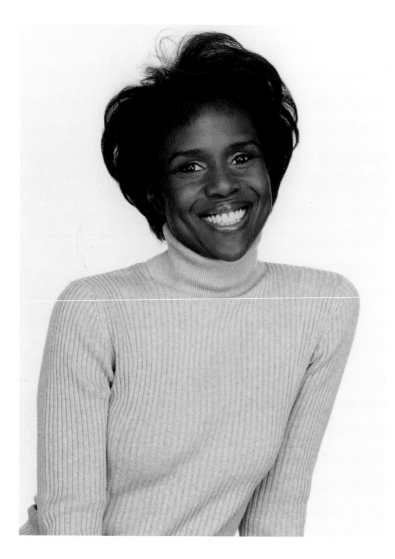

"I STILL FEEL TWENTY! AGE IS A STATE OF MIND. IT SHOULDN'T HAVE ANYTHING TO DO WITH WHAT YOU LOOK LIKE OR WHAT YOU FEEL LIKE. IT'S JUST A NUMBER."
—LAUREN, AGE 47 (RIGHT)

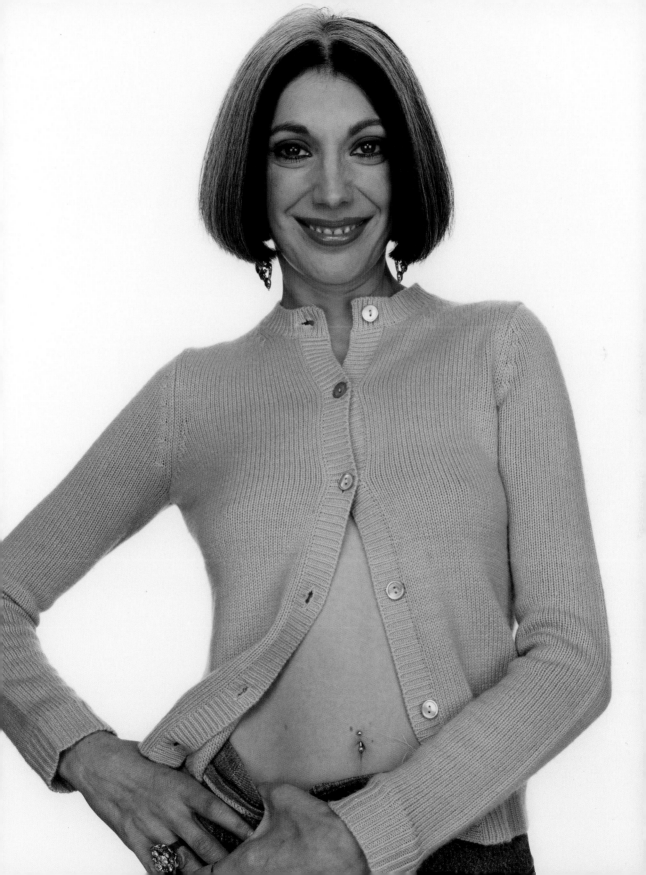

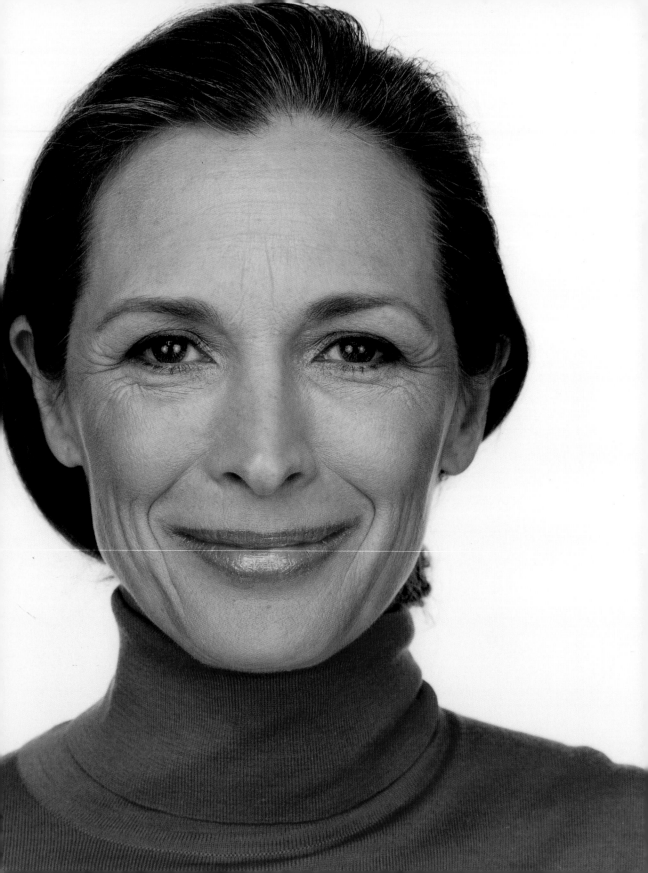

6 YOUR FIFTIES

To be in your fifties today is definitely different than it was years ago. Fifty used to be considered old. Now it's barely middle age. Celebrities in their fifties are proving that you can still look incredible (even without surgical assistance), be in amazing shape, and wear sexy styles. As a matter of fact, there's still plenty of time to get in shape in your fifties, even if you never had the time or motivation to do it before. It's not too late to start exercising, quit smoking, or start eating better.

Get that good haircut (if you've always had long hair, now is definitely the time to cut it above your shoulders). Invest in a few good clothes. If your kids are older, you'll suddenly have more time to yourself. If you're working, you're probably not still killing yourself to get ahead. This is the time to relax a little and feel good about all you've done in your life so far—and figure out where you want to go from here. In your fifties, more than ever, if you take care of yourself, it shows (and if you don't, it *really* shows).

In your fifties, more than ever, if you take care of yourself, it shows.

What you will notice in your fifties is that everything starts to fade— your hair color, your skin tone, your eyebrows. The solution is simple: Just add color. I think very few women look amazing with white or gray hair in their fifties. (But the ones who do should be thankful!) For most women, covering the gray is going to make them look younger, more alive. At this age, it can make the difference between looking like you're in your forties or in your sixties. (See chapter 21 for tips on choosing the right hair color and coordinating makeup to go with it.)

What You Need to Know Now
When it comes to makeup, you need a lot of knowledge. You are going to be wearing more color on your face, and to do that well, you need to know what you're doing. It doesn't work when it's overdone.

I see lots of women in their fifties who go overboard and wear too much makeup—it's almost like they don't want to see themselves. I suggest taking off all your makeup and really looking at yourself in the mirror. Look at what's good about your face, and don't look at what's "wrong." Start to appreciate what you see. Once you've done that, now you can look at what you don't like. Look at that feature and try to see what you can do to improve it or distract attention away from it. If you don't like your eyes, try to wear more lipstick or learn to line your eyes to make them look more defined. Remember that light colors lift, so use a bone eye shadow all over the lid and under your brows. Also, a brighter shade of blush (but be sure it still blends perfectly into your skin) will take attention away from fine lines around your eyes and give your whole face a lift.

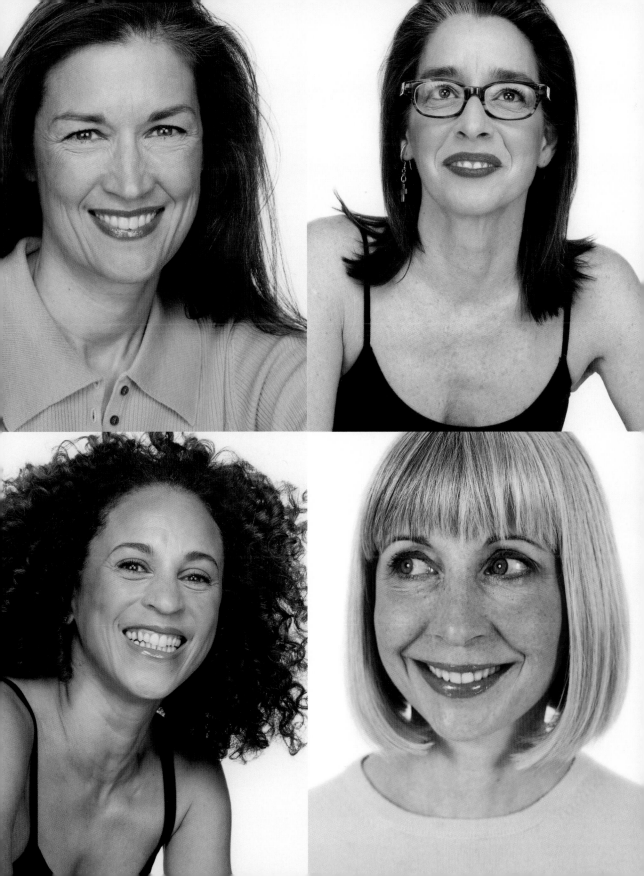

- **Extra-rich moisturizer:** Use it to make skin look fresher and lines less noticeable.
- **Creamy foundation:** Look for a moisturizing formula so that your foundation doesn't collect in lines and call attention to them.
- **Blush:** A bright touch will give your face a lift.
- **Lip pencil:** Use it to define lips and keep lipstick from feathering.
- **Eyeliner:** It can add definition back to eyes.
- **Eyebrow-defining shadow:** Don't be too heavy-handed; when in doubt, choose a softer shade.
- **Hair color:** This is often the key to looking younger at this age.

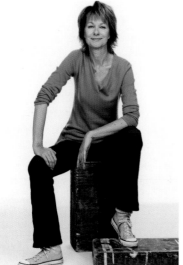 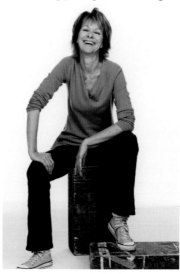

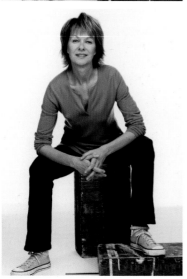 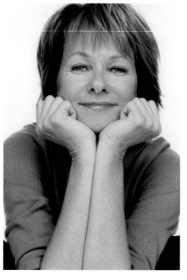

"WHAT I THOUGHT TWENTY-FIVE LOOKED LIKE, WHAT I THOUGHT FORTY LOOKED LIKE, WHAT I THOUGHT FIFTY LOOKED LIKE—ONCE I GOT THERE, IT WASN'T WHAT I THOUGHT IT WOULD BE AT ALL. IT TURNED OUT TO BE SO MUCH BETTER THAN MY EXPECTATIONS."
—SUSAN, AGE 50 (LEFT)

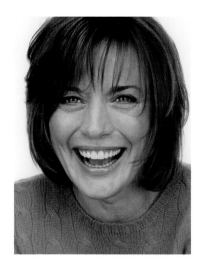

During and after menopause, you'll notice a change in your skin. As your body produces less estrogen, your skin (as well as your hair and nails) tends to get drier and the texture becomes rougher. Your face will look less dewy than it did when you were younger, so your makeup routine needs to start with making your skin look as smooth as possible. You can do that in layers—a rich moisturizer topped with a creamy foundation. And you need to keep all the colors you wear soft. Now is not the time to try wearing brown lipstick, but you can wear a more subtle pinky-brown, orangey-brown, or reddish-brown, plus a pink or apricot blush to give your face the color it needs to not look washed out.

You'll also start to notice in your fifties that your skin begins to lose definition—your lips might get lighter, your eyebrows are fainter, your eyes become less defined. You need to learn to line your eyes and your lips if you haven't been doing it before now. To define your lips and help keep the color from running, you need to apply a non-greasy moisturizer around your lips. Then use a pencil to line and fill in lips before applying a creamy matte lipstick. (See chapters 17 and 18 for more eye- and lip-defining techniques.)

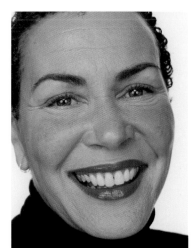

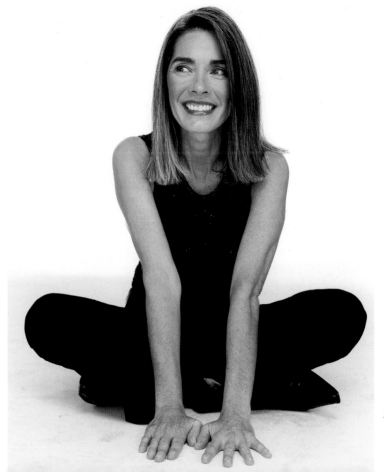

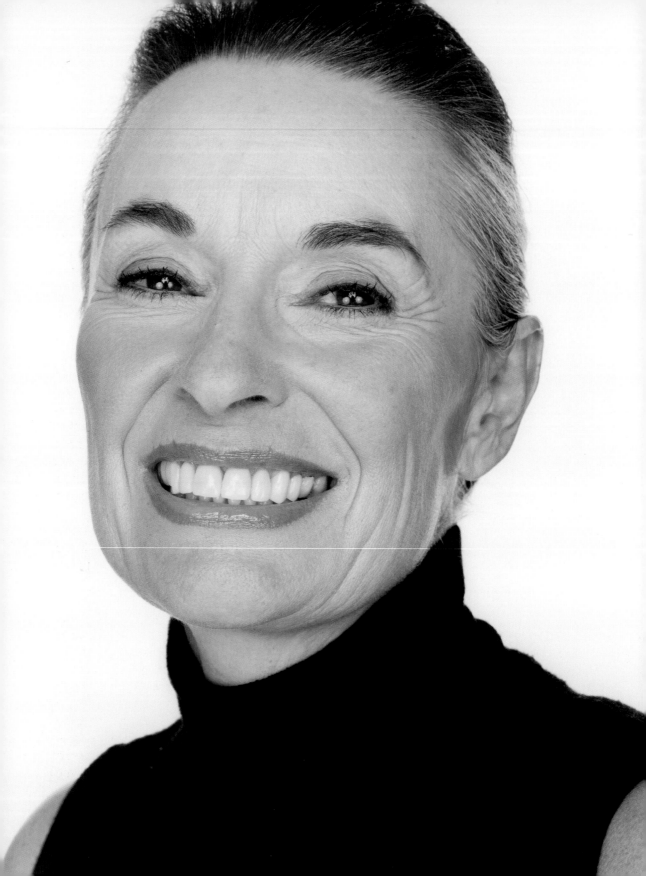

7 YOUR SIXTIES

Are you ready? Because this decade could be the big payoff. It's time for you to really start enjoying yourself and appreciating your life. Chances are, your children have left home, and you may have stopped working, so you have a little more time and money to spend on yourself. You might even have grandchildren, but that's no excuse to look like someone's little old grandmother! There are many ways to dress and do your hair and makeup that keep you young without making you look silly. And if you've taken care of yourself, stayed fit, and protected your skin, this can be an age when you look and feel incredible.

At this point in your life, looking good is really about the less you do to yourself—less, but of the right thing. There are so many women who, when they get older, think doing more is what will make them look better. But that often turns out to be too much—too much hair (overdyed, overstyled), too much makeup, and too much plastic surgery. I'd rather see women fresh out of the shower because they look ten times prettier untouched than after they've overdone it. I don't want to say that you shouldn't have plastic surgery because, honestly, I don't know how I'll feel when I'm in my sixties. But I do know that a little surgery—small nips and lifts—always looks better and more natural than having every inch of skin sliced and tucked. (See chapter 26 for more on plastic surgery pros and cons.) I admire and aspire to be like the women I see who wear their age with confidence and feel positive about themselves.

What You Need to Know Now
If you're not ready to go gray just yet, now is a good time to reevaluate your hair color. You may need to experiment, maybe trying something a little lighter than what you used to do. As you get older, your skin tone fades, so a hair color that used to suit you perfectly might suddenly look too harsh against your face. (See chapter 21 for advice on choosing the right hair color.) The same goes for the color of your eyebrows. Brows really fade in your sixties, and some women find that they seem to practically disappear into their skin altogether. The good news is that you'll no longer have to spend a lot of time with the tweezers, plucking and shaping your brows. The bad news is that you do have to spend the extra time defining them.

But be careful not to overcompensate by taking a black brow pencil and making them really dark. That's a big mistake I see a lot of women make. Just as with overly dark hair color, the contrast will look too severe. (See chapter 17 for brow-defining tips.)

Your face will need quite a bit of moisture in your sixties, so make sure all of your makeup is creamy. Start off with a moisturizer to plump up your skin. Then add a rich foundation and a cream blush that doesn't have powder in it. You could then layer with a pop of powder blush to add staying power. (In a pinch, you could even use a nice moisturizing lipstick as blush.) And since your skin thins out as you get older, you may start to notice that the area under your eyes looks darker. As always, the solution is finding the right concealer to both lighten and cover up dark circles. (See chapter 16 for makeup specifics.) That same concealer can be used to help hide age spots. Use a concealer brush to apply just a touch of concealer to the spot, and pat it on to blend. Add more if needed, and then put your foundation on over that. For lips that seem thinner than they used to be, the right liner will help. Don't use a dark liner (or too-dark lipstick either); it will look harsh and aging. Instead, use one that matches your lips' natural color exactly, or, to add more definition, use one that is one shade darker than your lipstick. Put your lipstick on; then line around the lips with the pencil.

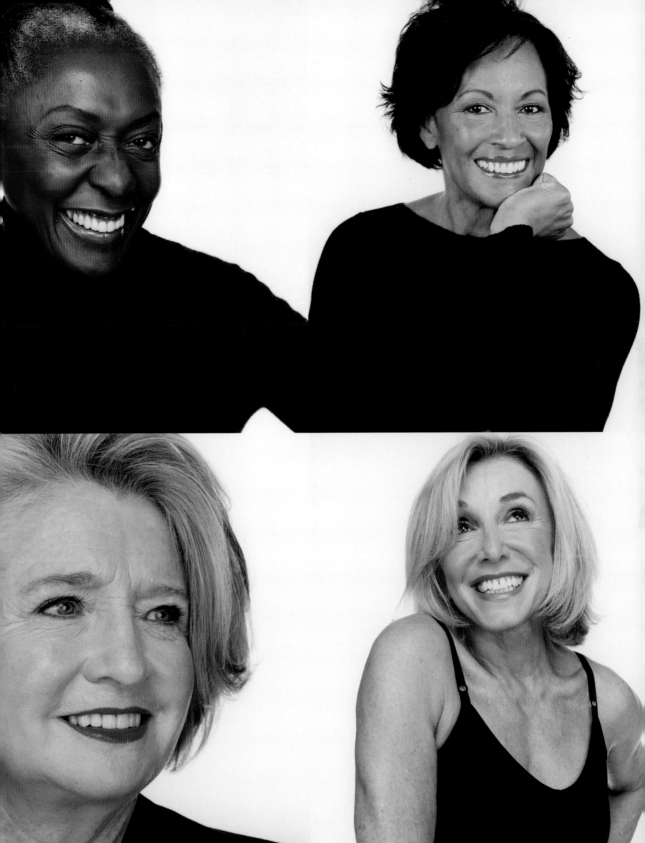

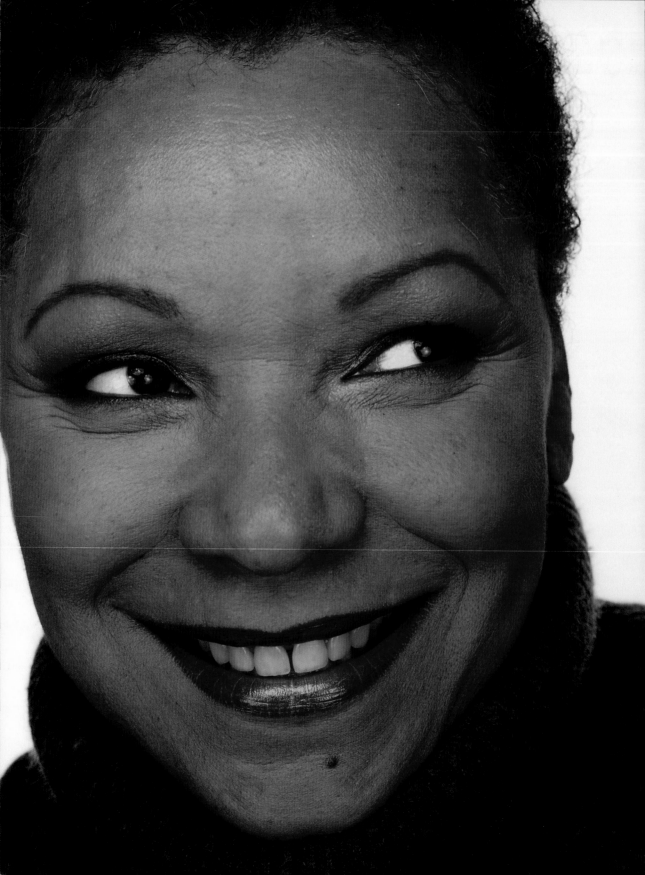

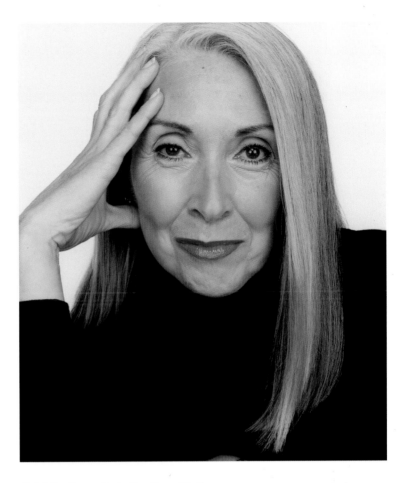

Bobbi's Essentials for Your Sixties

- **Hair color:** Lighten or brighten (don't darken).
- **A "no-curler" haircut.**
- **Skin care:** Use rich, creamy cleanser and moisturizer.
- **Creamy foundation:** It will glide over wrinkles, not settle in them.
- **Cream blush:** Make sure the color and consistency are right so as to blend easily into skin.
- **Concealer and concealer brush:** Use these for covering spots and under-eye circles.
- **Lip pencil:** Add shape and definition to lips.
- **Lipstick:** Use one with enough, but not too much, color.

"I FEEL THE MOST BEAUTIFUL NOW THAT I'M A 'SENIOR CITIZEN.' NOW THAT I'M OLDER, I APPRECIATE WHO I AM. I DON'T THINK THAT HAPPENS MUCH EARLIER IN LIFE."—AUDREY, AGE 65 (LEFT)

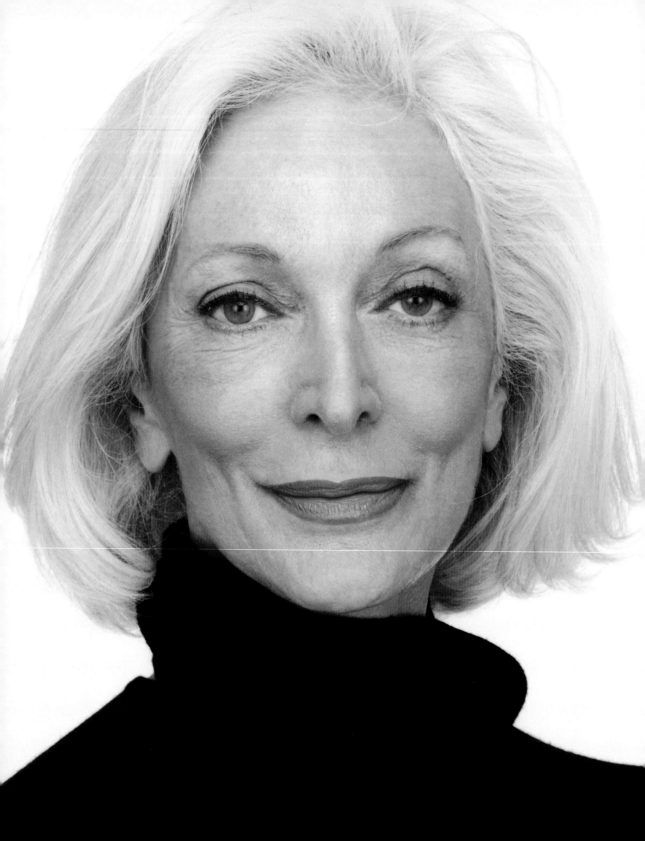

8 YOUR SEVENTIES... AND BEYOND

The biggest beauty secret for women as we get older is: Be active. It's very simple—just move! I don't care if you've been athletic all your life or never really did much—you need to walk, weight train, take yoga, play golf, whatever appeals to you. I promise it will make the biggest difference not only in how you feel but in how you look, too. It's going to be hard to make a huge lifestyle change at this point, but it's not too late to make subtle changes. I see women at the gym who are in their seventies who aren't necessarily in astonishing shape, but they look fantastic. They walk a little quicker and have more confidence than other women their age. These women are truly inspirational.

This is not a time to give up on your looks. But it is time, hopefully, to have made peace with them. I hate to think of women in their seventies and eighties going for plastic surgery. You've spent decades earning the face you have. Why try to change it now? That said, you still have the power to uplift yourself, make yourself look and feel better. It's amazing what just a little blush and lipstick can do for your self-esteem! You really don't need a lot of makeup when you're in your seventies or older. In fact, too much can look bad. You do need color, in shades that are flattering and pretty, but not too intense, because your natural coloring is very washed out. If you're still holding on to the same makeup colors you've been wearing since your fifties (or before), it's definitely time to update. Your skin, your hair, your brows have all changed, and you need new makeup to work with the new you.

What You Need to Know Now
Start with a rich moisturizer, a concealer, and then a little light foundation or even tinted moisturizer, a nice pink or coral blush, and rosy lipstick (or red lipstick if that's what you love, but steer clear of dark-brown tones). And you need to define your eyebrows because they do fade as we age. (See chapter 17 for tips.) Besides filling in your eyebrows, keep your eye makeup simple—just a bit of lid color to brighten your eyes (grays or heathers often look good). Cream or powder

formula is up to you; just be sure that whatever you choose isn't either too greasy or too dry. And if you wear glasses, you can probably get away with no eye makeup except for a light coat of mascara.

Lighting becomes increasingly important as we get older because your eyesight might not be as good as it was. My advice is to get a good magnifying mirror and really look at your face in daylight. It's a little scary, but it's the only way to make sure that you've gotten all those little hairs that sprout up in unwanted places (especially the chin). And good lighting will help ensure that your makeup looks right—that the colors work for you and that everything's blended properly.

Bobbi's Essentials for Your Seventies and Beyond

- **Rich moisturizer, oil, or balm:** Use this every day, even if you wear no other makeup.
- **Sheer foundation or tinted moisturizer (plus concealer if needed):** Heavy foundation can look masklike on older skin.
- **Blush:** Find a creamy formula that blends easily, plus a pop of powder blush to make it last.
- **Lipstick:** Creamy matte formulas moisturize but won't seep off lips.
- **Shadow:** Use it to fill in eyebrows.

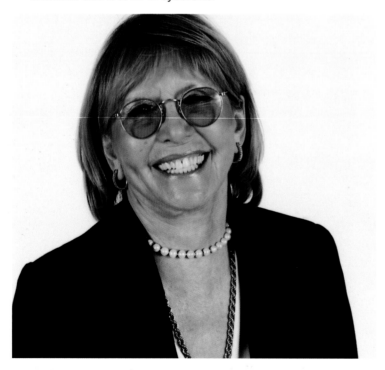

"THE BEST THING ABOUT BEING THIS AGE IS THAT I'M MORE FIT, HEALTHIER, AND STRONGER SO I AM ABLE TO PLAY WITH MY GRANDCHILDREN."
—THERESA, AGE 70
(TOP RIGHT)

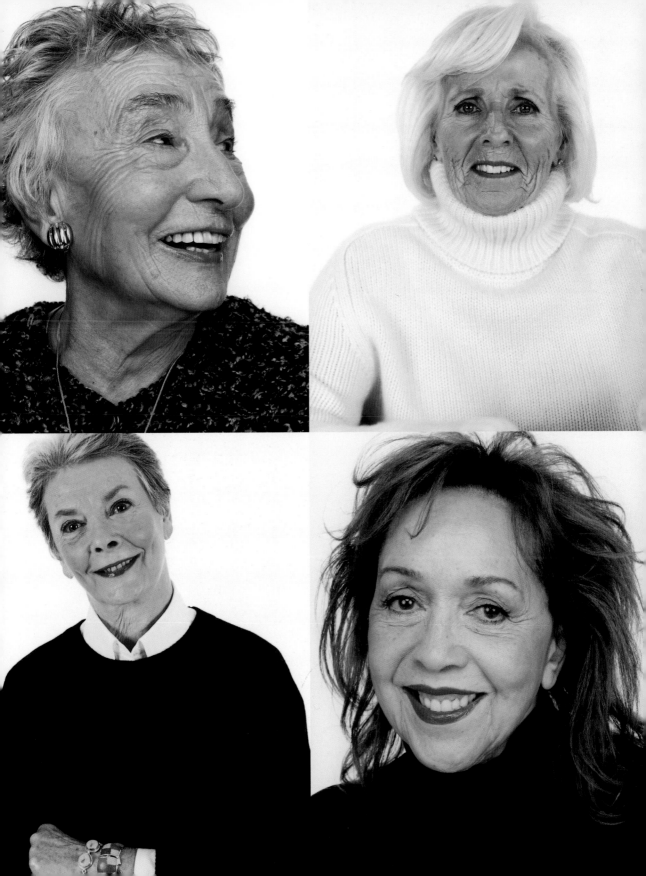

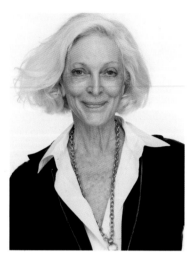

"I PROBABLY FELT THE MOST BEAUTIFUL AT BIRTH, AND THEN AT ABOUT AGE FORTY-SEVEN, WHEN I LET MY HAIR GROW IN WHITE. AND I PROBABLY HAD A BETTER BODY WHEN I WAS YOUNGER, BUT I DIDN'T FEEL THAT TERRIFIC."—CARMEN, AGE 70

Carmen before makeup (above) and after (below and opposite page).

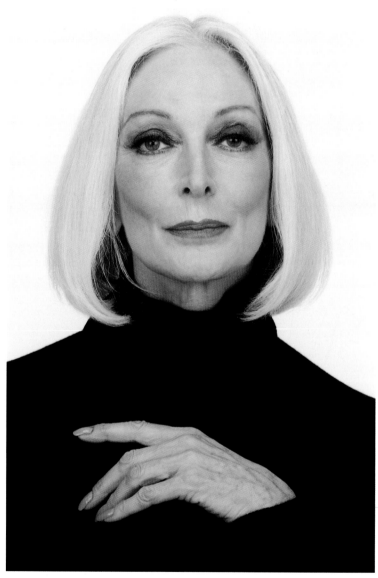

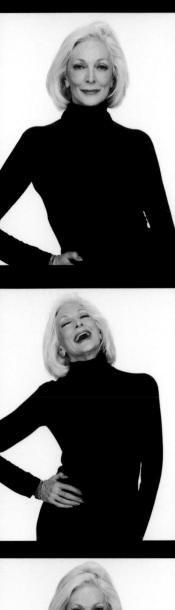
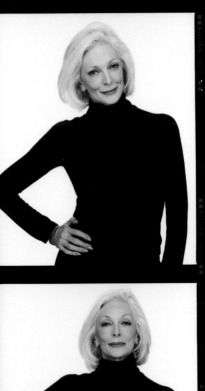

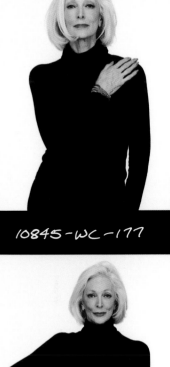

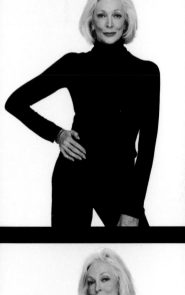
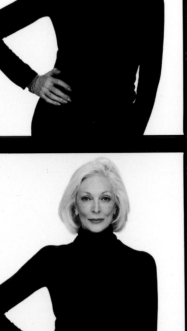
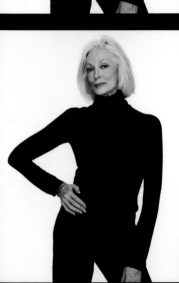
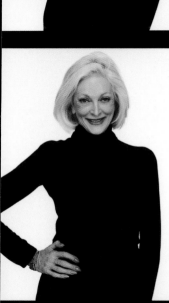
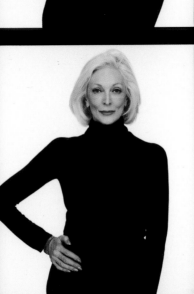

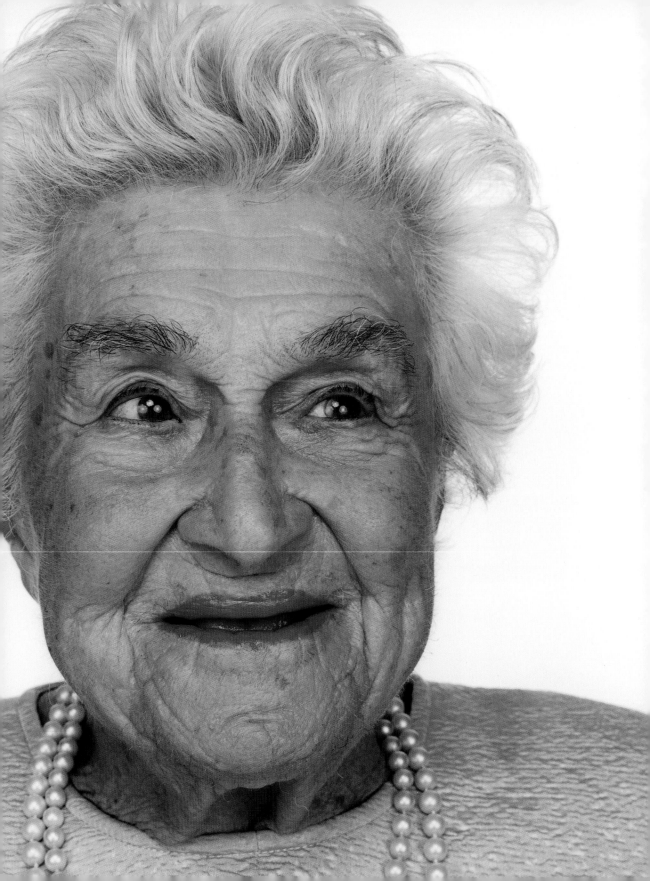

9 GETTING BETTER WITH AGE:
A ONE-HUNDRED-ONE-YEAR-OLD BEAUTY

Meet Dr. Lucia Servadio Bedarida. At the age of one hundred and one, she's still incredibly active, vibrant, and beautiful.

Born in Ancona, Italy, in 1900, Dr. Servadio Bedarida graduated cum laude from University of Rome Medical School in 1922 and became a surgeon. In 1923 she met her husband, a fellow surgeon, with whom she had three daughters. In 1939, they left Italy for Tangier, Morocco, where she practiced until 1980. At eighty years old, she retired and moved to the United States to be near her daughters.

"I had a wonderful mother and father and four brothers. They were very beautiful people, so I always felt in the background. That is probably the reason I studied medicine. To have something that was my own. I was always very good in school and liked to study, so I wanted to continue.

The best thing about being my age is the memories.

"I never really felt beautiful, but I think aging has made me better. I believe I am more beautiful at one hundred and one than I used to be. Even when I look at pictures from when I was younger, I think I am better now. I don't wear a lot of makeup—I just put a little color on my cheeks and some lipstick. And I always use powder. On my skin, I just use almond oil—the one you buy for cooking. Because when I was in Grasse, France, where they make all the perfume, I saw that the creams people pay a lot of money for are all made with almond oil. So I just use that.

"The best thing about being my age is the wonderful memories. I have had such a diverse life. And my life is still good. I live well. I am with my daughters; I still travel to see my family. My best memory of all is when I went hang gliding in the Alps. That was one of the best things I ever did in my life. It was unbelievably beautiful. Very exciting. I was ninety-seven years old then."

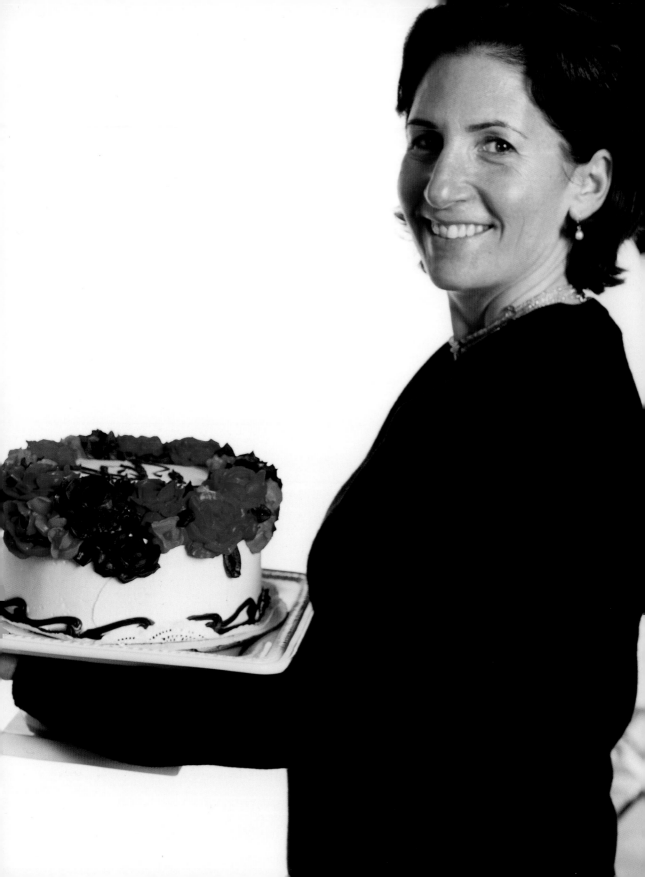

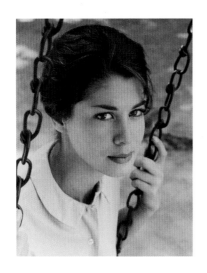

10 CELEBRATE!
A BEAUTY BIRTHDAY PARTY

What better way to celebrate a sixtieth birthday than by gathering together your closest girlfriends and getting pampered? That was my thought, so I put together a spa party at my house for my friend Rose. We did a mini yoga class in the living room and got manicures, massages, and, of course, professional hair styling and makeup application. Everyone wandered around in terry cloth robes and slippers (appropriately embellished with roses in honor of our birthday girl, Rose), eating, chatting, and getting beautiful. At the end of the night, we took group photographs of the ladies in their robes serenading Rose with "Happy Birthday." It was so much fun, and it made turning sixty look like the best thing that could happen to a woman!

"Every decade should be a celebration because it's an adventure, filled with new experiences."

"When I think about turning sixty, it's kind of shocking to me. My body may be there, but my brain is still in my twenties or thirties. It's a wonderful place to be because I still feel like I can do anything. Every decade should be a celebration because it's an adventure, filled with new experiences, new people. And when I look forward to turning seventy or eighty, I think of my life as a reductional state—like a sauce. You start to cook it down and get rid of all the fat and the surplus, and life becomes more simple. You reduce it down to the real essence of life."—Rose Cali

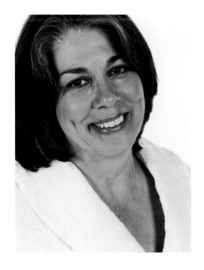

At left, birthday girl Rose Cali shows just how beautiful sixty can look. Above, Rose at eighteen.

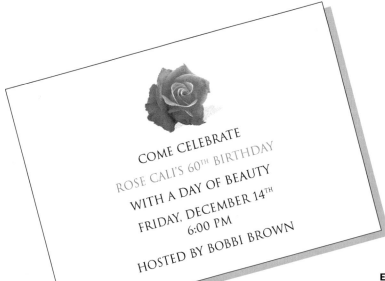

COME CELEBRATE
ROSE CALI'S 60TH BIRTHDAY
WITH A DAY OF BEAUTY
FRIDAY, DECEMBER 14TH
6:00 PM

HOSTED BY BOBBI BROWN

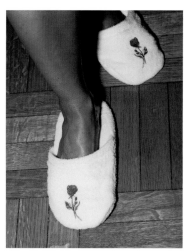

Even Yogi Berra (right) got into the spa spirit by getting a manicure.

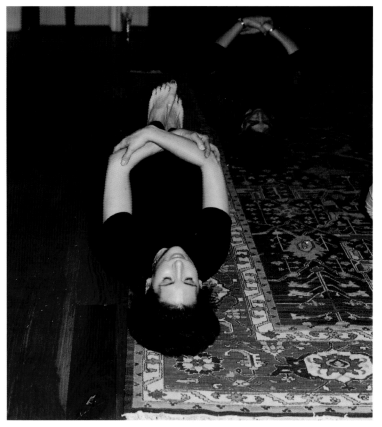

Party time: Yoga in the living room, beauty treatments, plenty of food, and rose-embellished robes and slippers in honor of Rose's big day.

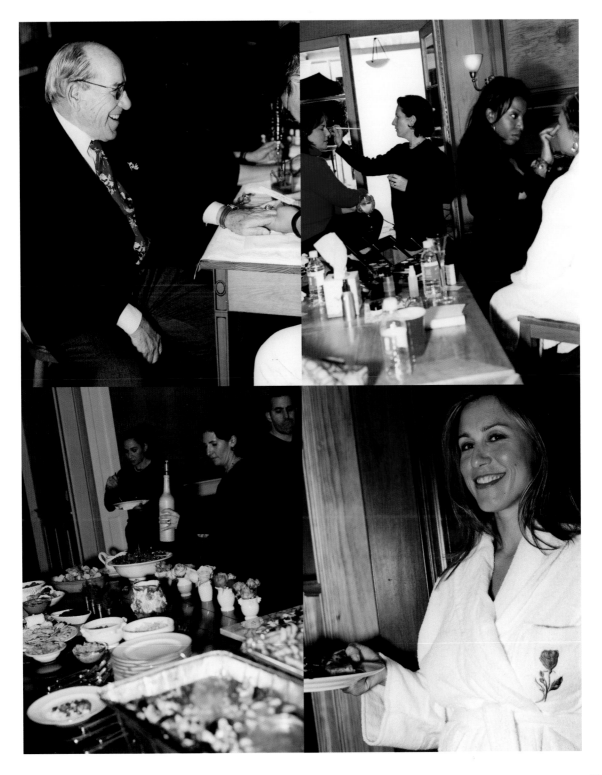

55

Bobbi's Favorite Beauty Gifts—to Give or to Get

- Cozy white terry cloth robe and slippers
- Lavender essential oil (to use in the bath or as scent applied directly to skin)
- Invigorating body scrub made with salt or sugar grains in a rich oil
- Soothing balm to use on lips, hands, feet, or face
- Gift certificate for a manicure, pedicure, or massage (especially if they do home calls)
- Anything that heats in a microwave to warm neck, shoulders, or feet

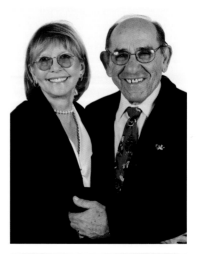

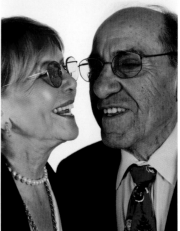

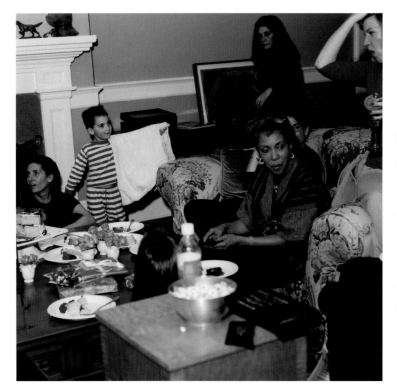

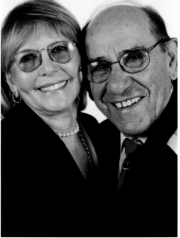

Yogi Berra and his wife, Carmen, mug for the camera.

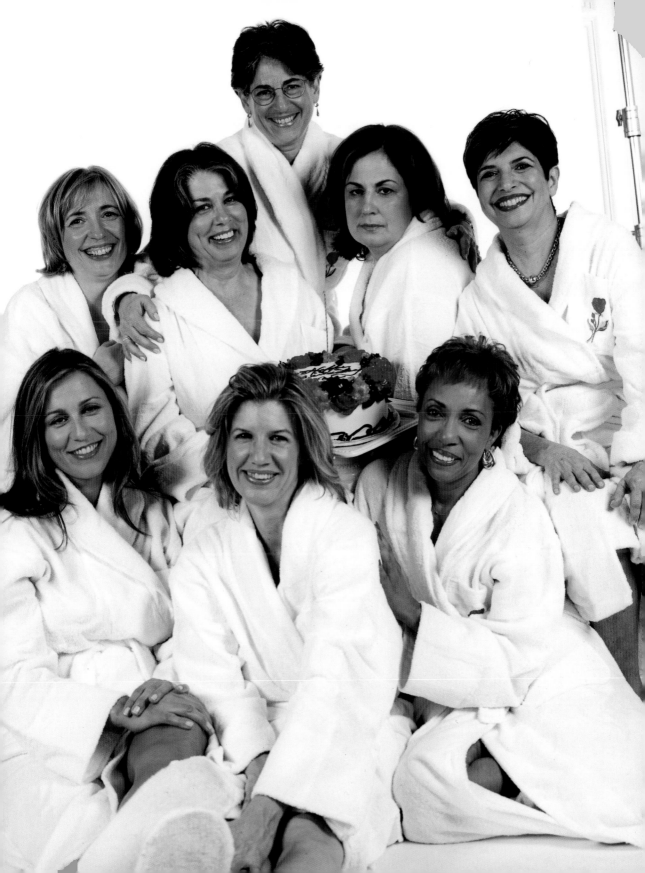

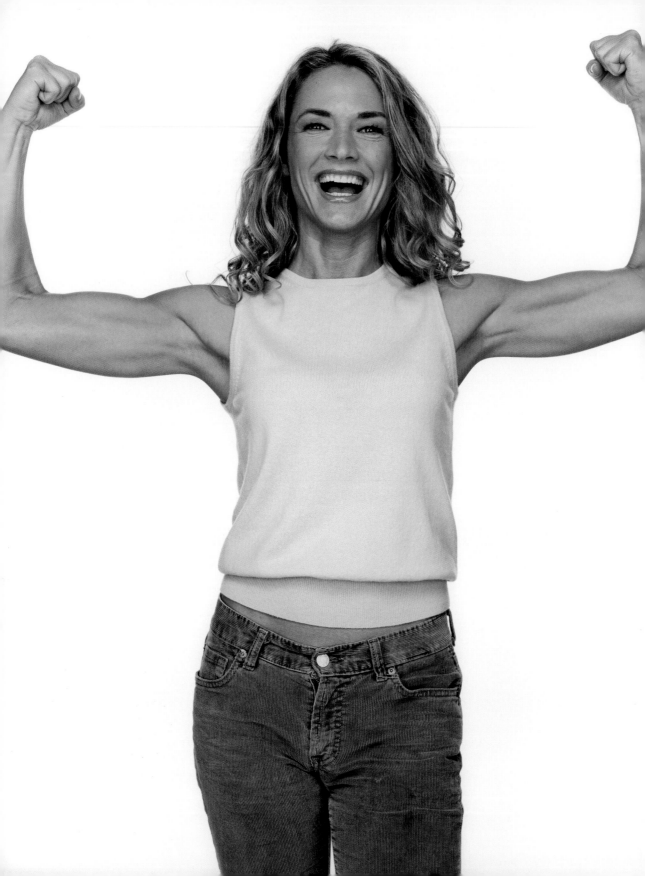

11 ANTIAGING MEDICINE:
HOW DIET, EXERCISE, AND YOUR LIFESTYLE CAN KEEP YOU YOUNG

My philosophy of beauty stems so much from how a person takes care of herself. As you age, whether or not you've taken care of yourself—eaten well, stayed active, not smoked, and protected your skin in the sun—makes a huge difference in your appearance. If you're healthy, you retain an overall youthful look and feel. And there's no question that when you feel good, you look better.

Two Ways to Look Old Before Your Time

Smoking. There is absolutely nothing you can do that will make you age faster than smoking. I think that smoking is probably the stupidest thing a person can do. Yes, I smoked when I was in college, but I quit when I was twenty-one, and I never looked back. People who smoke look like smokers. It's as simple as that. Their lips get gray, they get wrinkles around their mouths, their skin turns an ashy color, they smell bad, and, of course, they could die. If you do smoke, quit now. It's never too late to get back some of what you lost in terms of your health and your looks.

> Nothing you can do will make you age faster than smoking.

Sun. Too much sun exposure will also wreak havoc on your looks and, potentially, your health. That said, I don't believe in completely avoiding the sun. I do, however, strongly believe in protecting skin. We know too much now about the ozone layer and about the prevalence of skin cancer to take chances. Just as you wouldn't ride in a car without a seat belt, don't go in the sun without sunscreen. Wear a waterproof lotion (with an SPF 15 to 30) when you're outside, wear a hat whenever possible, and reapply after you sweat or go swimming. (In the city, you should have a minimum of SPF 15, and at the beach a minimum of SPF 25.) You don't have to hide; you just have to be smart. If you are a really outdoorsy person—a skier, surfer, golfer, whatever—your face will probably show the effects of the elements no matter how much you protect it. And that's fine because your healthy glow will shine through. You need to be extra careful about protecting your skin from skin cancer, but you should accept whatever lines you get as a result of your lifestyle and wear them with pride!

Eat to Live

I don't believe in being a fanatic about food, but I know I feel better when I eat better. And yes, it's hit or miss figuring that out. I've been on every single diet from the pineapple diet to Atkins. I lost weight and I gained weight, and the older I get, the harder it is to lose those last couple of pounds. But I feel like I've learned what's good for my body, what makes me feel good. It's about finding something you're comfortable with and that you can stick to.

But it's also about being realistic. If you generally eat healthfully, there's no need to deny yourself occasional treats. And when I travel, I just try not to worry about it too much. At home I eat as little white flour as possible. But believe me, if I'm in France, I'm going to have a croissant for breakfast, and if I'm in Italy, I'm going to eat pasta. Sometimes I come home from a trip and I've gained a few pounds. But I've had a great time and it was worth it!

Here are a few of the things that I've learned over the years that work for me.

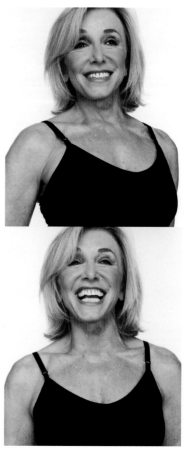

My stepmother, Lola Brown (above), and athletes Saskia Webber, Kym Hampton, and Dara Torres (right).

Try to have lots of:
Water
Lean protein
Vegetables
Brown rice
Whole grains

Try to have as little as possible of:
Caffeine
White flour
Processed foods/chemicals
Alcohol
Sugar

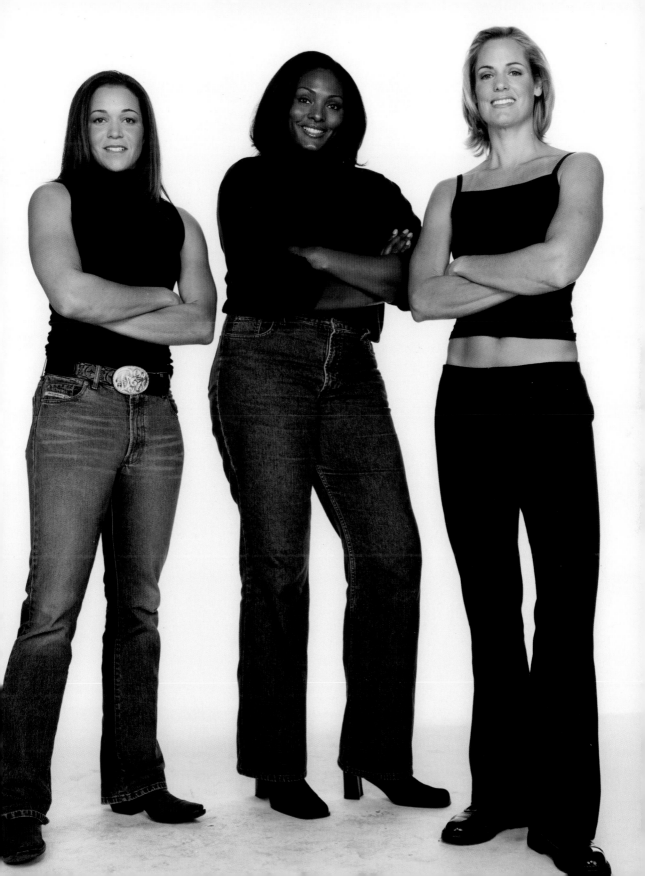

Of course, a balanced diet is essential at every stage of your life, but there are certain times when specific ingredients are even more integral to a healthy body.

Your twenties: Calcium. This is a prime bone-density-building decade—and nearly your last chance to do it (after age thirty-five, you stop building and start losing bone density). Be sure to get at least 1,200 milligrams a day. Good sources: skim milk, spinach, broccoli, cheese, and yogurt.

Your thirties: Folic acid. This nutrient is essential for the formation of fetal tissue, making it a must for anyone who is trying to get pregnant. You need to get at least 0.4 milligram of folic acid daily to help prevent birth defects like spina bifida. Good sources: enriched grains (pasta, flour, rice are all fortified with folic acid), green leafy vegetables, and beans.

Your forties: Fiber. If you haven't given your colon much thought up to now, it's not too late to start. Getting adequate fiber (you need 20 to 35 grams per day) will ensure that things run smoothly, keeping your colon clean and helping to prevent cancer. Fiber can also help prevent heart disease by lowering your cholesterol. Good sources: all plant foods—fruits, vegetables, and grains.

Your fifties: Calcium. Hopefully you never stopped getting enough calcium in your diet, but as you approach menopause, it's a good time to reevaluate your intake. With menopause, your body slows down its production of estrogen, which causes you to lose bone density. To hold on to all the bone you've got—and prevent osteoporosis—make sure you're getting at least 1,000 milligrams per day. Good sources: skim milk, spinach, broccoli, cheese, and yogurt, as well as calcium supplements.

Your sixties, seventies, and beyond: Calcium and antioxidants. Continue the calcium intake, and, in addition, take antioxidants. Examples of antioxidants are vitamins C and E, betacarotene, lycopene, and flavonoids, and their role in your body is to prevent potentially carcinogenic compounds from developing. A diet that's rich in antioxidants may help prevent some cancers and lower your risk of heart disease. Good sources: citrus and other fruits, nuts, seeds, yellow and dark green vegetables, and tomatoes.

Move It!

Staying active is probably the single best thing you can do for yourself to improve the way you look and how you feel. I didn't really start exercising until I was in college because when I was growing up, it

"I FELT THE MOST BEAUTIFUL WHEN I CAME OUT OF RETIREMENT AND STARTING TRAINING AGAIN."—DARA TORRES, SWIMMER AND OLYMPIC GOLD MEDALIST, AGE 34 (BELOW)

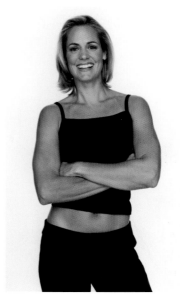

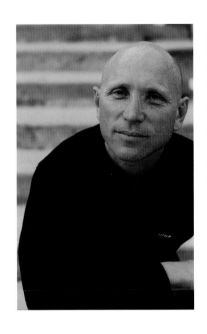

FITNESS TIPS FROM HOLLYWOOD'S LEADING MAN

Greg Isaacs, the director of the Warner Brothers Fitness Center and one of the fittest men I know, has whipped countless celebrities into shape. Here are some of his secrets.

- **Fitness is not an exact science**. There is no right or wrong approach. You need to find what works for you.

- **There are fundamental elements of fitness you need to incorporate into your life: cardio activity, flexibility, and strength.** The combination of all three will help you stay healthy, keep your body agile, and maintain your metabolism.

- **Jump-start your day with cardio.** You need to do something that elevates your heart rate for at least twenty minutes every day. Make it a daily discipline and include it in your schedule without thinking. (Just like you automatically go to work every day, you should also get some activity every day.)

- **Losing weight is as simple as energy in versus energy out.** If you burn off more calories than you eat, you'll lose. There is no big mystery and no need to eliminate food groups, try crazy diets, or starve.

- **Move your body every day.** Our bodies weren't designed to be sedentary, but our lifestyles have become increasingly so. The only solution is to figure out ways to fit more activity into your daily life—it doesn't have to be time at the gym; it could be walking the dog, taking the stairs, going dancing, or playing with your kids.

- **Find an activity you like to do.** So many people go to the gym and hate every minute of being there. In order to stick with an exercise regime, it has to be a fun part of your day. If it feels like a chore, try something else. Learn a new sport, do something you loved as a child (swimming, soccer), or try a fitness class that sounds intriguing.

- **Forget about the scale.** That should not be the way you judge yourself. Focus instead on how you look, how you feel, and how your body works.

- **Live a little.** There's nothing fun about going out to a party and not eating. Allow yourself a glass of wine or a piece of cake if you want. Just balance your nutrition and your exercise.

was mostly boys who played sports. I love seeing little girls now playing on soccer teams and taking tae kwan do—I can't think of a better way to empower a young girl. (So if you have a daughter, encourage her to be active by being active yourself.)

There are three major elements of fitness that you need to think about: aerobic fitness, flexibility, and muscle strength. I try to do something aerobic three times a week, whether it's running, doing the elliptical machine, or just taking a brisk walk with the dogs. For flexibility, I love yoga. I take Bikram yoga classes twice a week. And I'm a big believer in the importance of lifting weights. The older we get, the more crucial it becomes to have strong muscles.

Fitness May Be the Fountain of Youth

Weaker muscles, less stamina, more brittle bones, and a slower metabolism—these are just inevitable effects of getting older, right? Wrong. More and more, researchers are realizing that the changes people assume are the normal results of aging are really the result of inactivity and unused muscles. The solution: Exercise! Here's what it can do for you.

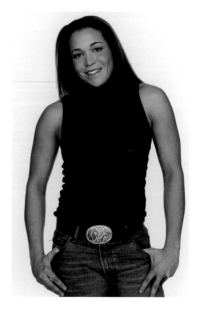

Soccer player Saskia Webber shows just how a good, healthy diet and exercise can be for your looks.

Boost your metabolism. In a true case of "If you don't use it, you lose it," your muscle strength declines tremendously as you get older. In fact, the average seventy-year-old has lost 40 to 50 percent of the muscle she had in her twenties. And since muscle tissue burns more calories than fat, having less of it slows down your metabolism, making it that much harder to maintain or lose weight. The good news: Strength training will slow down muscle loss, rebuild muscle that's already disappeared, and give your metabolism a kick-start.

Increase your stamina. As you get older, the airways in the lungs get less elastic, letting less oxygen into the blood. And the heart may be getting less blood flowing to it through the arteries, so your body is no longer as capable of performing aerobic spurts, such as racing for the bus, or endurance activities, such as skiing for five hours without a break. Again, the answer is exercise. Like any other muscle, the heart needs strengthening, and aerobic activity keeps it strong. Studies have shown that athletic women in their seventies have an aerobic capacity on par with inactive women half their age.

Better your balance. In your forties, balance starts to falter, and it can get worse as you get older. That is one of the reasons why so many older women fall, often breaking a hip or experiencing some other devastating injury. Take up activities that focus on improving balance, such as yoga or tai chi. At home, practice simple balance-enhancing tricks like alternately standing on one leg and then the other for thirty seconds while you brush your teeth or do the dishes.

Build strong bones. After age thirty-five, women typically lose 2 to 4 percent of their bone mass—more after going through menopause (because estrogen is a key ingredient in the bone-building equation). Aerobic activity and strength training both help not only to stave off bone loss but even to boost bone density.

Pump up your immune system. Exercise raises your heart rate, and that may be the secret to sending a surge of immune-boosting cells into the bloodstream where they are able to fight off potential threats. Improved circulation is another bonus of regular exercise, and good circulation helps carry those immune cells throughout the body. Studies have shown that staying active all your life can even help lower your risk of developing colon and breast cancer.

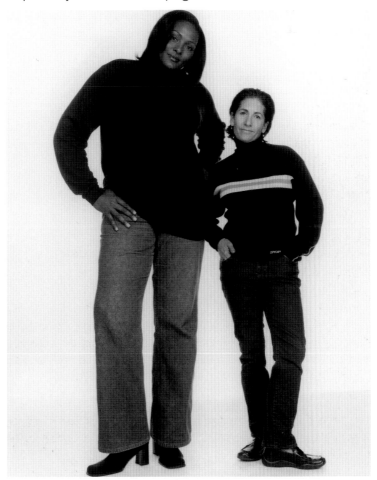

Proof that good things come in all sizes: basketball player Kym Hampton and me.

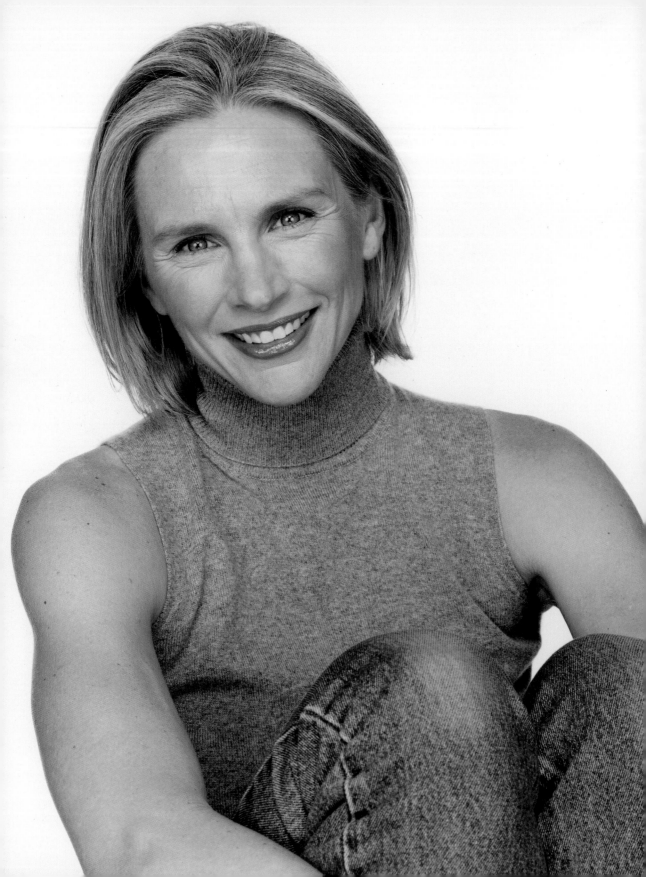

12 BEAUTY GETAWAY TO CANYON RANCH

I treated myself and my sister to a week at Canyon Ranch spa in the Berkshires of Massachusetts, and I loved it so much I wished I could move in. The surroundings were beautiful, the food was healthy and delicious, and I got to take so many invigorating walks, hikes, and exercise classes. But since we can't live at a spa—or even necessarily get to one at all—I wanted to pass on some of their wisdom, especially since their beliefs are very much in keeping with my own: It's all about commonsense health and wellness and how they affect both the way you look and the way you feel.

Bobbi's Best Tips from Canyon Ranch

I learned a lot about diet, exercise, and overall well-being during my stay at the spa. Here are a few of my favorite take-home lessons:

- **Get a refillable water bottle.** Make a habit of filling it up and carrying it around with you. Sometimes I add lemon, lime, or a splash of juice for extra flavor.
- **Load up on salad at every meal.** Chopped veggies add not only nutrients to your diet but also mega-fiber to fill you up (and clean you out). Canyon Ranch has the best no-oil salad dressing. They call it "Jet Fuel Dressing." Here's the recipe:

    ½ tsp. salt
    ½ cup red wine vinegar
    ¼ tsp. freshly ground black pepper
    1 tbs. sugar
    2 garlic cloves minced
    2 tsp. Worcestershire sauce
    1 tbs. Dijon mustard
    1 tbs. fresh lemon juice
    1 cup water

    Combine salt and vinegar, and stir until salt is completely dissolved. Add all remaining ingredients (except water) and mix well. Add water and mix well. Refrigerate. Best made the day before.
- **Pump up your normal workout!** Get your heart rate up by pushing yourself. Try interval training on the treadmill—alternating harder (uphill or faster) intervals with easier ones. (This was one of my favorite classes at Canyon Ranch.)

- **Keep learning and growing.** There is always room to change your life by keeping your mind open to new things.

Beauty Secrets from Canyon Ranch

- **Take charge of your hair.** It's not always the same, so don't treat it the same way every day, every season. If your scalp gets dry in the winter, consider a conditioning scalp treatment to add nourishment. At home, comb some conditioner through the hair and leave it on for a few minutes before rinsing out. Also, hair texture changes throughout your life due to hormonal shifts, pregnancy, and age-related pigment loss. Treat it accordingly by changing the products you use as your hair's needs change.
- **Exfoliate your skin.** Exfoliating rejuvenates the skin, smooths out tone, and even helps in the prevention of skin cancers. Use a grainy scrub, a washcloth, or a glycolic cream several times a week to help skin shed the dead cells.
- **Give yourself a mini-facial once a week.** For normal to oily skin, use a clay mask—it'll slow down oil production and help draw out impurities in the skin to unclog pores. Dry skin needs a nourishing, hydrating mask. And whatever you put on your face, bring it down to your neck—that skin needs attention, too.
- **Take care of your feet.** Be sure to use products specially formulated for feet—they have a higher concentration of ingredients than a product made for more delicate face or body skin. The best thing for softening feet is a glycolic foot cream (or better yet, a glycolic pedicure like they do at the Ranch!).
- **Mix up a skin-softening scrub.** Combine 1 tablespoon of salt or sugar with 1 teaspoon of body oil. Apply all over your body (don't scrub it on, but just let it roll over your skin), get in the tub, and let it rinse off by itself while you soak. For an even more luxurious

---

LAURA HITTLEMAN, BEAUTY DIRECTOR, CANYON RANCH, BERKSHIRES

"Beauty and wellness fit together. They're one unit. How we take care of ourselves as a whole person—what we eat, how we manage stress, our health—affects how we look. It's not about doing things to change yourself, like liposuction or zapping spider veins. It's about accepting who you are but working to maximize your health and your beauty and achieving a balance between inside and outside beauty. If you don't look good, you don't feel good. And likewise, if you don't feel good, you don't look as good. I used to say that people are looking for youth. But I don't think that's so much the case anymore. We're looking to take care of ourselves, feel healthy, and appreciate what we have."

experience, add a cup of powdered milk to your bathwater—the lactic acid leaves skin silky smooth.

- **Set the scene for relaxation.** Leave the TV off, hide the piles of bills and the to-do lists, light a candle, and tell the kids not to disturb you for ten minutes. Even a few minutes of uninterrupted time can do wonders for your mental health. Try to make time to pamper yourself once a week with a bath or an at-home facial.

Eat Yourself Beautiful the Canyon Ranch Way

Colorize your plate. Eat eight to ten servings of fruits and vegetables a day, including as many different colors as possible—red tomatoes, leafy greens, yellow squash, orange carrots, purple cabbage, citrus fruits, etc. Fruits and vegetables are rich in fiber; plus you'll guarantee a high intake of nature's powerful antioxidants, which not only work to fight cancer but also protect and renew the skin.

Go for grains. Whole grains, such as buckwheat and quinoa, are rich in skin-nourishing vitamin B.

Harness the power of protein. There's no need to go to the extremes of the popular (but not very healthy) high-protein diets, but sufficient protein is essential for the function of the immune system, as well as the health of the hair, skin, and nails. A general guideline: Divide your body weight in half and that's how many grams of protein you need as a minimum each day. Plant proteins (beans and tofu), fish, and lean meats are your best bets.

Eat healthy fats. Going fat-free (or even too low-fat) isn't good for you, and it's certainly not good for your looks. Not having enough fat in your diet can cause dry, flaky skin or dull hair and make skin more prone to inflammation. Look for monounsaturated fats (such as olive oil and avocados), nuts and seeds, and omega-3 fats (found in fatty fish and flaxseed).

Stay hydrated. Water is the forgotten nutrient and one that is so essential to beauty and well-being. Eating lots of fruits and vegetables (which have a high water content) is one way of adding more to your diet. And, of course, drink more water—and fewer dehydrating beverages that contain caffeine or alcohol. If your urine is clear, you're getting enough water. If not, drink up!

Clean up your diet. Move away from artificial sweeteners, food additives, and hydrogenated oils. (Yes, you have to read package ingredients—and pick the products that include mostly natural ingredients.)

KATHIE SWIFT, RD
NUTRITIONAL DIRECTOR,
CANYON RANCH,
BERKSHIRES

"I tell people that they should look at eating as an opportunity to enhance their natural beauty. Every time you sit down at the table, you have a chance to make yourself feel and look better—so use it wisely! We call it nutritional intelligence, and it's about knowing how the food you eat affects you both inside and out. Nutrients play a big role in the health of the body, and the health of the body is reflected in how the hair, skin, and nails look."

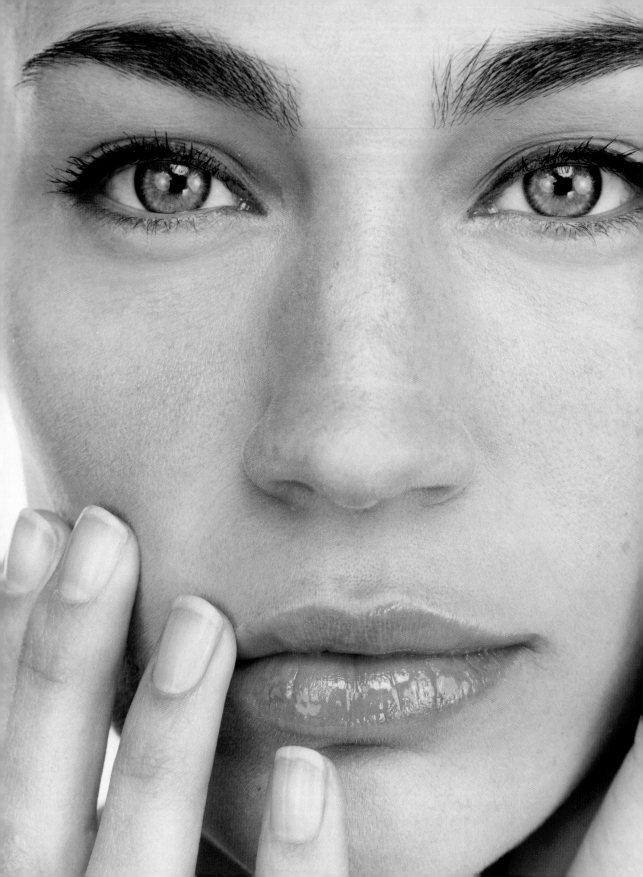

13 CARING FOR THE SKIN YOU'RE IN

I've met very few women who are satisfied with the state of their skin. It's either too dry or too oily or uneven in tone. Some complain about youthful breakouts and others simply think their skin looks old. I'm sorry to say that some of those things are just genetic, and there is no miracle product out there that will radically change the skin you were born with. What does help? Knowing your skin and using common sense when taking care of it. When you wake up in the morning, really look at your skin and what it needs. Don't just blindly reach for whatever you used yesterday because your skin could be drier, oilier, or more tired than it was yesterday. Being in control and knowing what to do is half the battle.

What Your Skin Would Tell You
It's no secret that your skin changes as you get older. The texture and tone you had in your twenties are completely different than what you have in your forties—and that's completely different than what you'll have in your seventies. Here's what to expect during each decade—and how to take the best care of your skin at every age.

Twenties. Barring bad acne held over from your teen years, your skin is at its absolute best in your twenties. Your skin is still manufacturing plenty of collagen, which keeps it elastic, supple, plump, and firm. **Skin care must:** Wash your face at least twice a day to help stave off excess oiliness, and take off all your makeup at night. And be sure to wear sunscreen every day to prevent future sun damage.

Thirties. This is when skin starts showing the early signs of sun damage—a few freckles or dark spots, fine lines around the eyes. And collagen production slows ever so slightly, meaning that skin starts to look less fresh. Exercising and keeping your weight stable will help skin stay taut—yo-yo dieting can affect the elasticity of the skin. **Skin care must:** It's all about hydration, both inside and out. Drink plenty of water, sleep with a humidifier (especially in drier climates), and moisturize the skin, especially the area around the eyes, which is drier, thinner, and ages the fastest.

Forties. By now, the environmental damage we accumulated in our teens, twenties, and thirties is written all over our faces—more lines, blotchiness, broken blood vessels, and brown spots. Collagen production slows down in your forties, meaning that skin isn't as elastic and may start to sag and look less firm. Smoking decreases the oxygen supply to your face, causing even more wrinkles. If you still smoke, it's not too late to quit and see improvements in your skin. **Skin care must:** Now is a good time to establish a relationship with a dermatologist and schedule regular appointments. Also, start using a moisturizer that protects skin from further damage and helps rebuild collagen.

Fifties. As you near menopause, you'll experience tremendous hormonal fluctuations—dry skin will get drier, and oily skin may get more oily. You will definitely need to double up on the moisturizer; use a rich, creamy one for dry skin or switch to an oil-free one if skin starts breaking out. **Skin care must:** Get your moles checked. This is a good time to step up your vigilance—see your dermatologist for annual checks, and keep an eye on them yourself to look for any that change size or shape.

You've earned the face you have now, so wear it proudly.

Sixties, seventies, and beyond. Skin care is really all about maintenance at this point. Continue all the good habits you've gotten into—keeping skin clean and well hydrated, wearing sunscreen, getting your moles checked regularly. **Skin care must:** Relax about your looks! Now is not the time to freak out about every line or brown spot. You can get the thing that really bothers you fixed if you want or just learn to live with it. You've earned the face you have now, so you might as well wear it proudly.

A BOBBI REMINDER

IF YOU STILL SMOKE, IT'S NOT TOO LATE TO QUIT AND SEE IMPROVEMENTS IN YOUR SKIN.

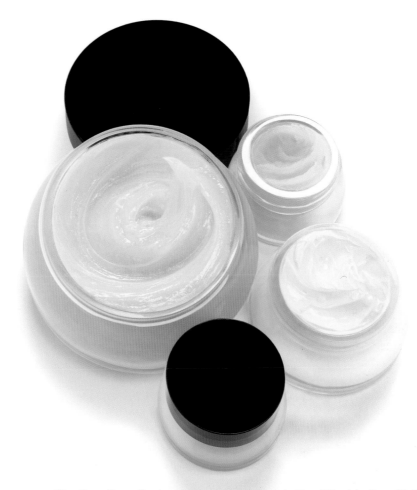

The Bare-Face Basics: What You Absolutely Need Next to Your Sink

Cleanser. You really have to try a cleanser to know if you are going to like it because so much of what makes you like a cleanser is how it feels, whether you like the amount of lather, whether it smells good, and if the package looks nice sitting on your bathroom sink. I don't believe in using soap on your face because it really strips the skin. If you have oily skin, you should use a gel cleanser, which will cleanse your skin and limit oil without stripping the skin. Dry complexions should stick with a cream cleanser. Some lather, while others are more like a lotion that can be rinsed or wiped off skin to clean and add moisture to skin. Ideally, you should have two different cleansers: one for the days when your skin is a bit oilier than normal or needs extra cleaning and one for days when your skin is a bit drier than normal.

Toner. To me, a toner is an optional step in your daily routine. If you have very oily skin or if you wear a lot of makeup, it can be a good way to clean away anything your cleanser has left behind. (If you feel like you need toner to remove residue left behind by your cleanser, switch cleansers. The right one should rinse off clean.) And be careful to choose an alcohol-free toner that's not stripping your skin. If your skin feels tight and dry after washing, skip the toner that day.

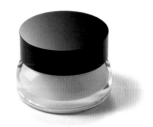

Moisturizer. This, in my opinion, is the most important step in caring for your skin. When your skin isn't well moisturized, it looks dull, tired, and older than it is. Ideally, you should have more than one moisturizer on hand so that you can pick the one most appropriate for your skin's condition as it changes from day to day and season to season. An oil-free formula is perfect for adding moisture to oily or blemish-prone skin without causing greasiness or clogged pores. A hydrating cream is truly a cream—just oil and water—with no added goodies. It's perfect for extra dry or sensitive skin. Somewhere between the two is a moisturizing lotion that's heavy enough to hydrate normal skin but won't make it look greasy.

Sunscreen. An SPF lotion is essential anytime you'll be heading outdoors—and that includes walking from the bus stop to the office. Wear an SPF 15 to 30 every day, and try to find one that's not sticky under your makeup. For skiing or the beach, step up to a heavy-duty waterproof sunscreen (SPF 30 to 50).

Eye cream. Eye cream is key because most regular moisturizers aren't gentle enough (especially if they contain SPF) to use on the delicate skin around the eyes. You should have a light eye cream to put on in the morning before you apply concealer, and as you get older, you might want to add a rich, gooey one for night. There are also lots of eye creams on the market with special ingredients—such as vitamin C and K—that claim to help erase dark circles and reduce puffiness. They may help, but I've yet to find a miracle.

A La Carte Items: Pick Just the Ones That Are Right for You

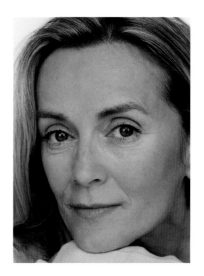

Face-cleansing wipes. I'm a big fan of things that are easy, and these wipes are a great alternative for those nights when you're just too tired to bother with your usual routine. I don't think they are good enough to use exclusively on a regular basis, but they're a fast way to take off your makeup and clean at least some of the day's grime off your skin before bed.

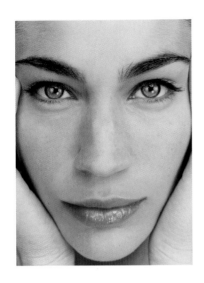

Shine-control lotion (for oily skin only!). Apply before foundation to keep skin oil-free and makeup smooth. This is great for combination skin—use it on the T-zone (forehead, nose, and chin) and use moisturizer on drier spots, like the cheeks.

Masks. All skin types can benefit from a mask once or twice a week. Clay masks are great for cleaning out pores. A hydrating mask will help rejuvenate dry skin. And glycolic acid masks—which exfoliate the skin—can help oily skin get rid of clogged pores as well as help diminish fine lines on all skin types. You can buy glycolic masks over the counter that contain up to an 8 percent concentration (these shouldn't be left on for more than five minutes or they can irritate skin), or a dermatologist can do an in-office treatment using a stronger version (often called a "glycolic peel").

Serums. These are a luxury because they are expensive and aren't essential to caring for your skin. They are concentrated liquids that deliver potent doses of vitamin C or other skin-nourishing nutrients. If you use one every day, it will help your skin have a tighter, smoother appearance. It usually takes about four weeks to notice a difference. Just remember that serums don't replace moisturizer—they have to be used with a cream on top.

Balms. Thick, viscous, but not oily, these super-rich moisturizers are great for softening dry patches on face, feet, hands, and body, and even for smoothing down hair (apply a bit to palms and run lightly over your hair).

Exfoliating agents. It's important to slough off the dead skin cells on your face so that they don't clog pores, making skin either break out or look dull. But you need to be very gentle with your face—don't treat it like a pot that you're scrubbing with Brillo. It's best to use a scrub that's made especially for your face (it will be less abrasive than ones made for the body) or even just rub gently with a soft facecloth. Leave the harsher scrubbing tools—loofahs, sea sponges, and Buff Puffs—for your body.

Face oil. This is a soothing and healing treat for dry, parched skin.

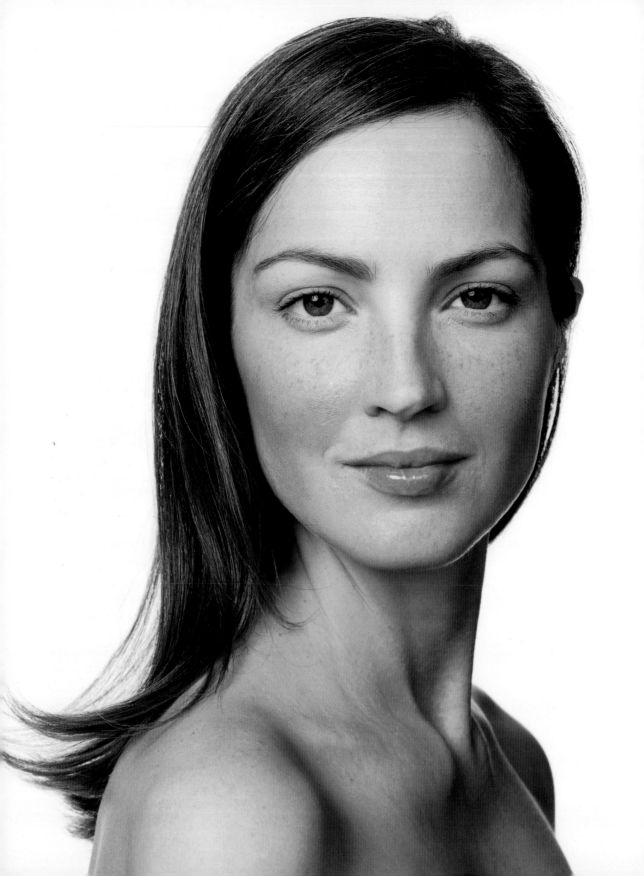

Looking for a Miracle?

There are dozens of creams and potions out there that claim to work magic on the skin—eliminating lines, plumping up texture, and smoothing out tone. My opinion is that there are no miracles! But I do think that many of these products can make subtle differences in your skin tone and texture and in how pronounced the lines on your face look. I'm also a great believer in the placebo effect—if you think these creams are making you look better, you *will* look better (and feel better about the way you look). Here are some of the most common ingredients to look for.

Alpha-hydroxy acids (AHAs). These are naturally occurring acids in fruits and milk that are used topically to diminish fine lines. They help speed up skin's natural exfoliation process, which is helpful for both unclogging pores that lead to breakouts and improving the texture of aging skin. One of the most commonly used AHAs is glycolic acid.

Antioxidants. Ingredients such as vitamins C and E, betacarotene, green tea, and grapeseed extract are all antioxidants. They protect the skin against environmental hazards—molecules called free radicals that damage skin cells and lead to premature aging of the skin.

Retinoids. These powerful vitamin A derivatives (like Retin-A and retinol) have been proven to fight acne as well as reverse signs of aging. They also build collagen to help skin look firmer and more elastic. The downside: They can be irritating (you need to build up a tolerance gradually) and may cause skin to become extremely sun-sensitive.

Kinetin. This is a plant-derived antiaging agent that helps smooth and restore skin's radiance.

Coenzyme Q. An antioxidant that exists naturally in the skin and may help lessen premature signs of aging.

Copper. A factor in elastin synthesis, copper may help restore skin's firmness and elasticity.

Skin Care from the Neck Down

Skin is the largest organ in your body, covering every inch of you—even those parts you tend to forget about, like your heels, elbows, and back. Caring for the skin on your body is, for the most part, a lot simpler and more straightforward than caring for the skin on your face. But it needs to be done—so be careful not to neglect everything from the neck down. And yes, the skin on your body (like the skin on your face) will start to sag as you get older. The only thing you can do about it is keep your muscle tone up. Unfortunately, no amount of weight lifting will make a sixty-year-old arm look like a thirty-year-old arm, but it will help tremendously.

Body skin care can be summed up in two words: exfoliate and moisturize.

Exfoliating options. Getting rid of dead skin cells will keep your legs and body from getting that dry, scaly look. Use a loofah, a washcloth, or a body scrub (they have grains in them, like salt, sugar, or synthetic particles, that gently rub away dead skin) in the shower, and pay special attention to rough areas like elbows, knees, and heels.

Body oil. The easiest way to moisturize your entire body in a hurry is with oil. I keep a plastic bottle in my shower, and right before I get out, I put some in my hands, rub it all over my body, and then carefully towel off. I'm not a big fan of dry oil—it doesn't sink in, so it doesn't moisturize as much.

Body lotion or cream. Either works, and the only rule is the richer, the better!

Perfumed body lotion. I love using perfumed body lotion to moisturize my skin after a shower. The scent is really light, it stays on all day, plus you're accomplishing two things at once (moisturizing and putting on perfume). Sometimes I put a touch of perfumed lotion on my hands and run it over my hair—it leaves a light hint of scent in my hair and smooths it out as well.

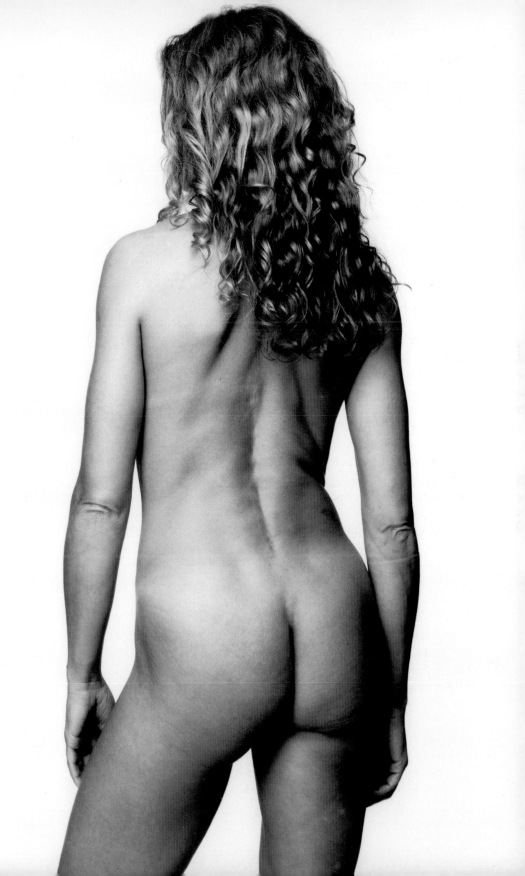

Feet. Getting a professional pedicure once a month is the best way to get your feet in top shape, but even with that you need to keep up the care on your own. Keep a pumice stone in the shower and give rough spots (especially heels) a quick rub every morning. An AHA cream will help feet slough off dead skin too. And moisturizing will also make a huge difference—do it as soon as you get out of the shower; at bedtime, slather feet with Vaseline (over the AHA cream).

Cuticles. The skin around your nails can easily become dry and ragged, especially in colder, drier weather. The only solution is to moisturize like crazy—hand cream, oil, Vaseline, or cuticle cream rubbed into and around nails several times a day.

Bumps on backs of arms. Not exactly a rash and not pimples, these little bumps plague many women. I find that the only thing that really helps is to exfoliate arms gently in the shower (even just rubbing with a washcloth will do) and then apply some moisturizer or body oil right afterward.

Body breakouts. If you have a serious problem with acne on your back or chest, you should consult a dermatologist. For more occasional breakouts, try a shower scrub that contains salicylic acid—it will help to slough off dead skin that clogs pores as well as control oil production.

Age spots or discoloration. AHA lotions used regularly can help lighten dark patches on the skin. You can also cover them with a combination of foundation and concealer. (See chapter 16 for tips.) If you want to erase them completely, you might need to try a chemical peel or laser resurfacing. (See chapter 25 for options.)

Spider veins. These aptly named creatures (which appear most often on the legs and face) are caused by the dilation of small groups of blood vessels close to the surface of the skin. They aren't harmful and usually aren't painful, but they can be unattractive. If they bother you to the point where you want to get rid of them, the best solution is a procedure called sclerotherapy. This consists of injecting a saline solution into the vein, causing it to collapse and become scar tissue that is then absorbed by the body. Another option is laser surgery. Depending on how superficial the problem is, a laser can be used to

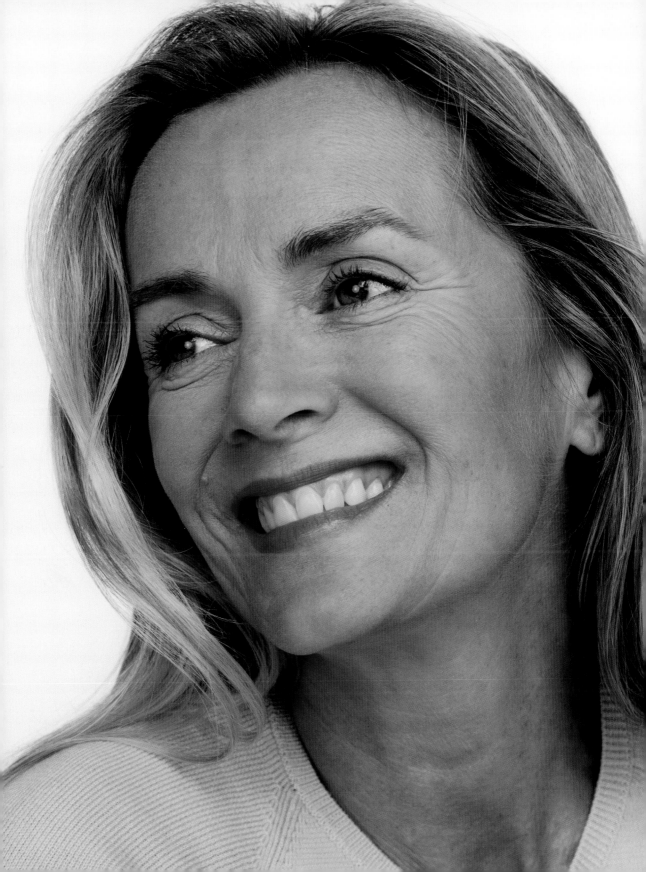

zap and destroy the veins. Unfortunately, neither option will prevent new spider veins from forming.

Cellulite. Contrary to what many manufacturers would like you to believe, there is no cream that can rub away cellulite. These fat deposits that typically appear on the hips, butt, and thighs are best controlled with diet and exercise (although genetics make some women more susceptible no matter what they do). The best result you can hope for from any of the anti-cellulite potions is a temporary smoothing of the skin surface.

Hair Removal

There are several methods of removing hair that's growing where you don't want it, and which you choose is really just a matter of personal preference. And the older you get, it becomes almost funny where those unwanted hairs show up—like on your chin or the sides of your face. My favorite hair removal methods are shaving (the cheapest, fastest, and most convenient) and waxing (for hard-to-shave areas). Here, the pros and cons of them all.

Shaving. You can't beat shaving for convenience. You run a razor over your legs or under your arms while in the shower, and that's the end of it. The trick is making sure your skin has a lot of moisture on it before you start shaving. Wash with a really creamy soap first, and then use a foamy shaving cream. I think a good men's razor is the way to go (the disposable ones are okay in an emergency but don't give you a great shave). To avoid a fight, never use your boyfriend's or husband's razor! Or if you must, at least replace the blade immediately. Best for legs, toes, feet, or underarms. Never shave anywhere on your face.

Waxing. Yes, it hurts. But it's quick, lasts a few weeks, and gives the smoothest results in areas like the bikini line that can get irritated by shaving. The downside is that you have to let the hair grow in a bit before you can wax it again (which is why I don't like this option for my legs). The bikini area is tricky, so I'd recommend letting a professional do it. Brazilian bikini waxes—an extreme job that takes off almost all the hair (ouch!)—have become very popular. You can do small waxing jobs, like your upper lip, at home. There are several at-home wax options: one that heats up in the microwave (very convenient), one that comes in a block that you need to heat in a small pan on the stove, or no-heat strips (check drugstores and beauty supply stores for options). If you decide to do it yourself, be very careful: Never leave the room while you're heating the wax, and test it on your wrist to make sure it isn't too hot before you apply it. Dry the skin by dusting it with baby powder. Apply wax in the direction of the hair growth and then pull it off in the opposite direction in one quick motion (like you'd take off a Band-Aid). Then wipe the area with witch hazel to soothe and disinfect. If any hair becomes ingrown (common when waxing the bikini area), don't pick or it might become infected. Try applying Tend Skin (available at drugstores and beauty supply stores) or rubbing gently with a washcloth in the shower to loosen ingrown hairs. Best for bikini line or upper lip.

Laser. A low-energy laser is used to target a large area of hair follicles. The energy passes into the follicles and immediately disables them. What will determine the number of treatments required is the size of the area that's being treated and the density of the hair growth. The process isn't a guarantee that hair will never regrow, but it does seriously stunt growth. Best for women with light skin and dark hair (the laser can affect the pigment in darker skin).

Depilatory. I find these a little too messy and a bit stinky to use on a regular basis. But they do work in a pinch when you don't have time for a bikini wax. Best for upper lip or bikini line.

Tweezing. This is great for shaping brows and for getting rid of those rogue hairs that pop up on our chins as we get older. (See chapter 17 for tips on tweezing brows.) Best for small areas or single hairs.

Electrolysis. This is the only permanent method of hair removal, but that permanence doesn't come quickly or painlessly. It can take years of regular appointments to get rid of the hair on your upper lip—making this too expensive and time-consuming for many women. Best for small areas like the upper lip or sides of the face.

To avoid a fight, never use your boyfriend's or husband's razor!

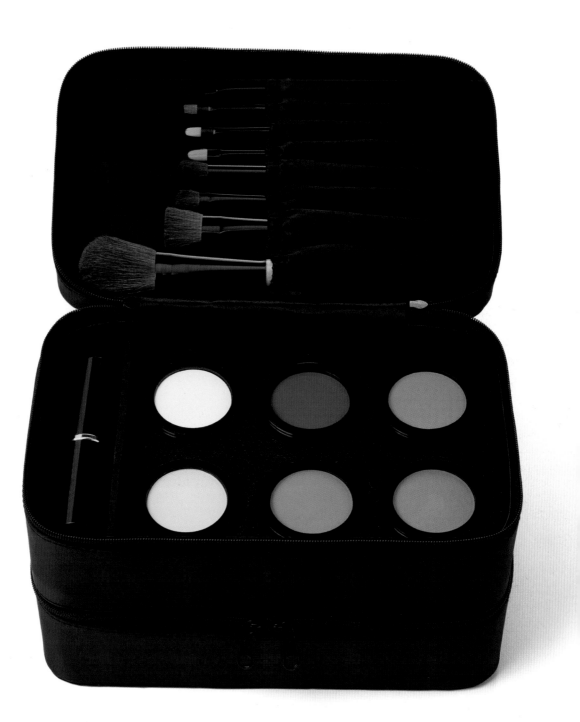

14 YOUR TOOLBOX:
BRUSHES, SPONGES, AND MORE

As with any other job, putting on your makeup requires the right tools—in this case, that means a selection of brushes, sponges, and puffs that make your makeup easy to apply and flawless-looking. You don't have to spend a fortune on brushes for every area of the face, but having at least a few good ones can make all the difference. Even a makeup minimalist should invest in a couple of essential tools. Here they are, plus optional items for those women who want a really complete tool kit.

The Brush Essentials
It's easy to tell a good brush from a bad one. The bristles should feel soft against the skin—never scratchy or rough. Whether the bristles are made of natural or synthetic hairs isn't as important as how they feel. A lip brush or concealer brush, which needs to be stiff enough to apply a thicker, creamier product, is actually best when made of synthetic material. But your eye shadow, blush, and powder brushes need to be soft and fluffy so that they spread out over your skin. Try out the brush by running it across the area of the face it's designed for to make sure it feels right. And also test the strength of the bristles: Run your hand over the bristles and make sure they do not come out in your hand. Practice using it and see if you like it. The handles need to feel comfortable in your hand. If the handle is too long and unwieldy for you to maneuver, look for a brush with a shorter handle.

Generally, the brushes you'll find in makeup artists' lines are going to be the best and probably worth the extra money. If you can afford them, good brushes will make a difference in how your makeup looks and how easily you can apply it. But you can also find good brushes for less money if you really look in drugstores, beauty supply shops, or even art stores. Of course, no one at the art supply store is going to help you and say, "This is a really good eye shadow brush." So do your homework and check out the expensive makeup brushes; then go see if you can find something equally good elsewhere for less. And if the brushes you buy don't say on the handle what they're for, label them yourself. Take the brush that the salesperson said is for lining your eyes, stick on a little piece of white adhesive tape, and write "eyeliner" on it.

A great set of brushes will last you a long time if you take care of them. As a general rule, you should clean your brushes every three to five months. But how you clean them is even more important than how often you do it. Wash them with a gentle soap—baby soap, baby shampoo, or Dr. Bronner's liquid soap. (Brush cleaners that contain alcohol can dry out the bristles.) Don't fill the sink up with water and soap and toss the brushes in because if they soak in water for too long, they will start to fall apart. Instead, take a drop of liquid soap in the palm of your hand, wet the brush, and then wipe it around in your hand. Be very gentle—even the best brushes are fragile. Once all the bristles are covered in soap, it's time to rinse. The trick is to make sure you get all the soap out (that's why something like baby shampoo is good because it doesn't lather too much and rinses easily). Whatever soap you use, a little of the scent will remain, so you might as well choose one you like. After the brushes are rinsed completely clean, squeeze out the excess water with a paper towel or clean towel and then air-dry them by letting the bristles hang off the edge of a counter. The bristles shouldn't touch anything; otherwise they may start to smell mildewy and dry funny, with the bristles pushed to one side.

Bobbi's Three Must-Have Brushes

1. Blush brush: Get rid of the one that came with your blush. I've never seen a good brush that came with a blush. Those are usually short and narrow, and you want one that's rounder and wide enough to cover the apple of your cheek (but not as wide as a powder brush that would cover too much of your cheek).

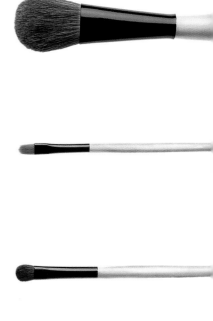

2. Eyeliner brush: There are several choices of brushes you can use for your eyeliner. A thin, flat brush (with either straight or slightly rounded bristles) is my favorite. It helps you draw a line that's not too thin or too wide, it works with wet or dry eyeliner, and it's good for the top or bottom lid. A thin, pointed brush is the smallest eyeliner option and will help you create a very thin, deliberate line along your top lid. A brush that's cut on a diagonal is a bit thicker and is best for applying a smudgy sweep of shadow liner.

3. Eye shadow brush: This brush should be soft and fluffy and should spread out easily when it touches your lid. It should be big enough to cover about a quarter of your lid at a time but small enough that you still have enough control to place the shadow properly.

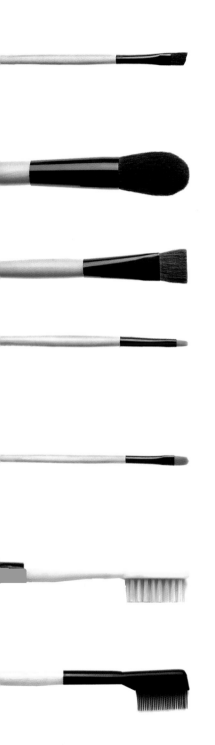

- **Eyebrow brush:** This is an optional brush that may become more essential as you get older and need to use shadow to define and darken your brows. A good eyebrow brush is slanted, and the bristles are hard and a bit scratchy. Use it to apply the shadow to define your brows (but never use this brush for anything else; it's too hard and will hurt your skin).

- **Powder brush:** I think that a velour puff is actually the best way to apply powder because it helps smooth the powder evenly all over. You can use a puff to apply the powder and then take a brush just to wipe off the excess. This should be your biggest brush, with wide, soft bristles that are either rounded or cut to point (great for getting around the eyes and nose).

- **Wide eye shadow brush:** This is bigger and fatter than your basic eye shadow brush, and you use it when you want to sweep a single base color over your entire lid.

- **Lip brush:** The bristles should be firm but bend easily as you apply it to your lips. Lip brushes come in different shapes—flat, angled, or pointy. I find the angled ones harder to use and prefer one that's somewhere between pointy and flat. A lip brush that retracts or has a cover is great for keeping in your purse.

- **Concealer brush:** You can definitely use your fingers to apply concealer, but a brush makes it easier to get more concealer exactly where you want it. If you have bad dark circles under your eyes or age spots you want to cover, then this is a brush you need. The end is tapered so that you can get concealer into hard-to-reach areas, like the inner corners of the eyes and around the nose. A good concealer brush is similar to a lip brush but a bit thicker, longer, and softer. The bristles should be firm but not too hard because you will be using this brush on the delicate skin around your eyes.

- **Brow grooming brush:** This is different than the brush you use to apply shadow to your eyebrows. This brush is also made from stiff, scratchy bristles, but they go straight across like a toothbrush (in fact, a toothbrush could work in a pinch). You use this to brush your brows upward and to corral any stray hairs into place.

- **Eyelash comb:** I never use one, but some women like to comb their eyelashes to separate them after applying mascara. If you are careful with the way you brush on your mascara, you can skip this extra step.

Beyond Brushes

Makeup brushes are obviously going to be your biggest beauty tool investment, but there are a few other items you might want to have on hand to help apply your makeup. Disposable sponges are great. Buy the ones at the drugstore that come in little wedges—get a big bag of them and don't try to make it last forever. When a sponge gets dirty, throw it out and take a new one. (I'm pretty fanatical; I use them one time only.)

You can buy powder puffs at the drugstore too, but the better-quality ones, which are more expensive, are well worth it (all the makeup artist lines make them). You can hand-wash it or throw it in the dishwasher to clean it and make it last longer. If you like using sponge eye makeup applicators, I recommend buying a bag of disposable ones and replacing them often. It's more sanitary, and your shadow colors will look truer if you apply them with a clean sponge.

And while curling your lashes isn't essential, eyelash curlers will help open up eyes and make lashes look more lush (with or without mascara). Look for one that feels comfortable in your hand, holds lashes firmly, and doesn't tug at the hairs.

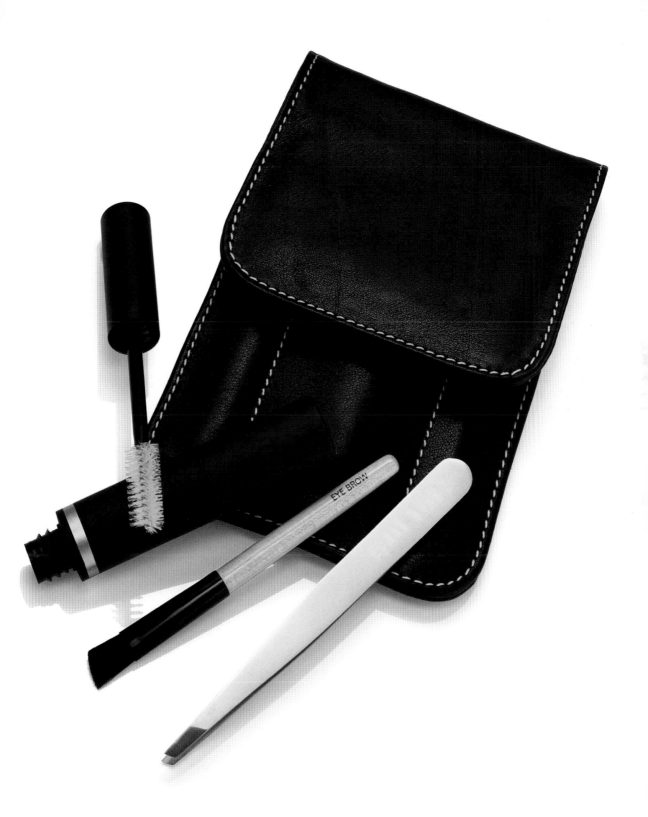

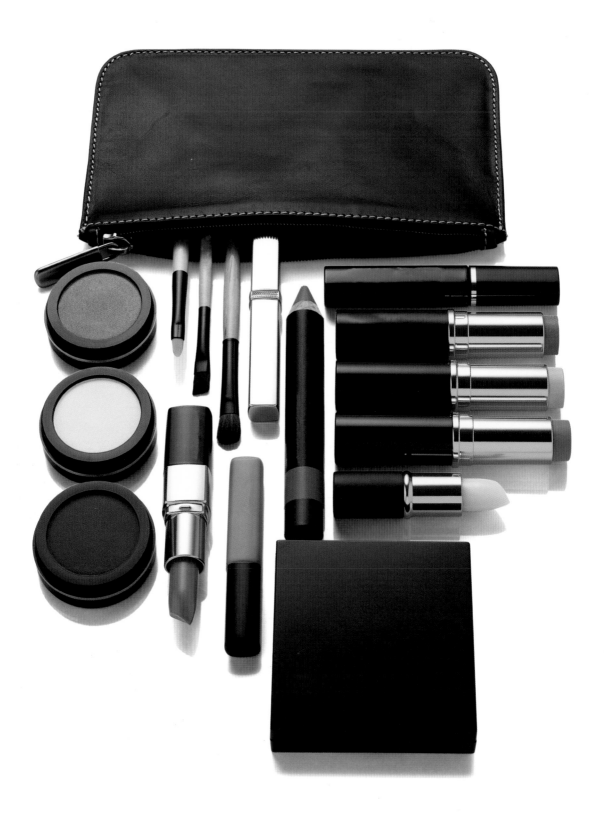

15 PURGE, THEN SPLURGE:
WHAT TO KEEP, WHAT TO TOSS, WHAT TO BUY

First You Purge

Why bother organizing your makeup? Because it makes it easier to get ready. Just like it's easier to find an outfit to wear to work in the morning when your closet isn't crowded with outdated clothes, doing your makeup is simple and quick when you open the drawer or cabinet and everything you want to use is right there in front of you. Put everything in its place, and I promise that you'll be able to put your makeup on in five minutes. Searching for your favorite eye shadow or cleaning up foundation that spilled because the bottle cap is broken wastes valuable time. But if you take some extra time to organize, toss out old stuff, and repackage broken things—do it twice a year—you'll save yourself time every day. You'll feel great and in control.

To start, empty out your makeup drawer, bag, or cabinet, and take a good look at everything that was in there. Get rid of anything that's broken, leaking, or generally a mess. If you can, transfer the product into a new container. Liquid foundation can be poured into a new bottle, and lipsticks with broken caps can be sliced off and put into a palette or even those day-of-the-week pillboxes they sell at the drugstore. Lip and eye pencils that are missing caps should go in clean Ziploc bags. But broken powder compacts, blush, or eye shadow really should be tossed. If it's your absolute favorite shade—and the company doesn't make it anymore—then keep it in a Ziploc bag. Otherwise, toss it and treat yourself to a new one.

The next step is to get rid of anything you've had for at least two years and haven't touched. Maybe it was some trendy color you loved in a magazine but hated when you got it home. Or the texture never felt right on your skin. Or the formula made you break out. Whatever the reason, get rid of it. Put all that stuff that you've barely—if ever—used in a box to donate to people who may be able to use it, such as a theater group or a women's shelter.

Now that you've cleared away the messy stuff and the stuff you know you're never going to wear, it's time to turn a critical eye to your basics. Start with your foundation. If you have five or six different ones, that is a bad start. You really need only two at the most. (See chapter 16 for tips on finding the right one.) Open each one up and smell it. If any have a weird odor—or if the consistency seems funny— that's your cue to put it in the trash. Foundations do go bad after a year or so, even sooner if they are stored in the sun. Now that you've weeded out any that are past their expiration dates, grab a mirror, apply a swipe of each of the remaining foundations to your cheek, and check out the results in natural light. Only the ones that disappear into your skin are worth keeping. Ideally, you'll end up with one that matches you perfectly now and another that'll be a perfect match in six months when it's a different season and your skin tone is slightly lighter or darker.

Next, take a look at all of your lipsticks. I find that this is the product many women tend to overbuy. If you're one of those women, chances are you're about to discover more lipsticks than you ever thought you had. Hopefully, you've already tossed the ones you haven't worn in two years and transferred broken ones into clean palettes. Look at what's left and be realistic about how many you really will wear. The ones you've been saving to go with that special dress you also never wear can probably go, as can the impulse buys that you didn't really love when you got them home. Lipsticks can be mixed to make a better color out of two that aren't quite right. Put them in a palette and experiment if that's something you enjoy. I'm a believer in only having things that really work—not things that take work to make look right—but that's up to you. Next, do the same analysis on your eye shadows and blushes.

As long as you've got all your makeup out, now is a good time to do a little maintenance work. Use a Q-tip dipped in alcohol to clean off your makeup cases, replace old sponges and powder puffs, and check to see if any of your makeup is past its prime. Take a good look, especially at your mascara because that has a really short shelf life—only about three to six months. I find it helpful to write on the tube when I bought it so I don't accidentally keep an old one hanging around too long. You can also tell because the consistency gets dry and flaky. And if you have a habit of putting on your makeup in the car (which I think can be a great time-saver in the morning—provided you're not the one driving!), be aware that storing your makeup in the glove compartment or in a place where it gets a lot of sun can seriously shorten its shelf life.

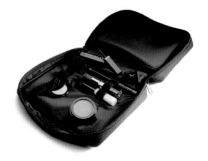

Once you clean your drawer and take a look at the makeup still there, you'll probably have about a fifth of what you had before. But the way I look at it, you actually have more because everything there really works for you. There are a million different ways you can organize your makeup, depending on the space you have. You can use a silverware organizer to slip into a drawer, lucite boxes to stack on a vanity, or cups to place your brushes and pencils in. Hopefully, you'll be so inspired by this exercise that you'll take another hour to organize your medicine cabinet (what are all those old prescriptions for anyway?) and even your clothes closet.

This is also a good time to clean out, restock, and reevaluate the contents of the makeup bag you keep in your purse as well as your travel cosmetic kit. I like to have a bag with duplicates of makeup basics to carry with me all the time. That way I always have what I need for midday touch-ups or reapplying if I go right from work out to dinner. If any of your at-home makeup didn't survive your purge, you'd better check your on-the-go bag, too. It's even more essential that whatever you keep in there is perfect—the exact right color of concealer and foundation, pressed powder, a soft, pretty blush, and your everyday lipstick. I also keep a travel kit packed and ready to go at all times—with small bottles of my essentials like cleanser, moisturizer, and shampoo. Take a look in there, and refill or refresh anything that's empty or old—that way you'll be ready to head off for the weekend at a moment's notice.

Expiration Dates

No, it doesn't last forever. Here is a general timetable for your makeup's life span:

Foundation	**12 to 18 months**
Concealer	**1 year**
Powder	**2 years**
Mascara	**3 to 6 months**
Lipstick	**12 to 18 months**
Lip or eye pencil	**1 year**
Eye shadow	**1 year**
Powder blush	**2 years**
Cream blush	**6 months to 1 year**
Moisturizer	**12 to 18 months**
Eye cream	**1 year**
SPF lotion	**1 year**

Then You Splurge

Now that your makeup has been thoroughly weeded out and well organized, you may notice a few glaring holes. Did you suddenly realize you don't own a single lipstick you really love? Or that none of your foundations are a perfect match? Well then, it's time to go shopping!

I think the biggest complaint women have about buying makeup is that they feel so pressured by the salespeople to make a purchase. So the first thing to remember is to know your rights. You don't have to buy anything in any situation. If you've just had a makeover, it's often better to say, "Let me think about it," and walk away. You may need time to get used to how you look if you're trying something new, such as a brighter lipstick or a more neutral eye shadow. Try to go outside and look at yourself in natural light. If you decide you like what you see and still love it when you catch a glimpse of yourself in the mirror an hour later, go back and buy whatever products they used. On the other hand, if you put on a lipstick at the counter and instantly know it's perfect, then by all means buy it on the spot. But do not buy anything that you don't love just because you feel guilty that the salesperson spent time with you. Every time I hear a woman say, "She made me buy it," I envision a woman sitting on her hands while the salesperson steals her credit card. I want to empower women to feel more in control than that. If you buy something, it's because you chose to buy it, so it should be something you actually want to own.

If you're still undecided, another option is to ask for samples or trial sizes of products you aren't quite ready to commit to. This is especially useful for skin care, and many companies will give you minis that last up to a week. That way you can see how your skin reacts before you invest in a big bottle of a cleanser or moisturizer.

Department stores certainly aren't your only option for makeup shopping. There are drugstores and places like Target or Wal-Mart that carry all the drugstore lines. It can be hard to buy anything that you really need to try on (like foundation) at these stores, but they're great places for picking up trendy colors cheaply or things that you don't really have to try first, like nail polish. At the other end of the spectrum are the makeup specialty stores. It can be a lot of fun to go to a freestanding store of a brand. It's like going to a freestanding store of a fashion designer—you get to see the entire line displayed just as the makeup artist envisioned it. Plus, I do think the makeup artist lines really have the best foundations. The tones are much truer to skin tone than even the better department store brands. And Sephora has created an entirely new way to shop for makeup. Those stores are a makeup addict's dream come true! With so many brands in one place—and pressure-free try-ons—it's the ultimate place to do comparison shopping.

Shop Talk: A Store-by-Store Guide to What to Buy Where

TYPE OF STORE	THE PROS	THE CONS	THE BEST BUYS
Drugstore	It's convenient and inexpensive.	You can't try before you buy, making it hard to choose the right foundation, concealer, or powder.	Nail polish, mascara, skin care, and possibly eye pencils—although it's better if you can feel these first.
Department store	Most of the sales-people at the counters are trained makeup artists, and you can try products on before you make a purchase.	Sales pressure—some of the counter sales-people will make you feel like a criminal if you test products or ask questions and don't buy anything.	Foundation, concealer, powder—anything you really need to try on first.
Freestanding store of one makeup line	There is a better selection of a brand you already know you like, without the tough sales talk of most department stores.	You might not find everything you need in one makeup line.	Great colors of lipsticks and eye shadows as well as true-to-skin-tone foundations and concealers—all are available.

Buyer Beware

You do have rights at the makeup counter. Here's how to exercise them:

- You are under no obligation to buy a thing after a makeover, unless something was specifically stated before the makeup artist began working on you.
- You can ask for samples and trial sizes of products, whether or not you're making a purchase.
- If you get a product home and think it's past its expiration date (the texture is off or it smells funny), bring it back for a refund or replacement.
- Before buying products you can't try (as is the case at most drugstores), find out what the store's return policy is. Some places will let you bring back unsatisfactory products for exchange.
- Hold your ground! If all you really want to buy is a lipstick, don't allow yourself to feel pressured into buying the matching nail polish or whatever else the salesperson is trying to push.

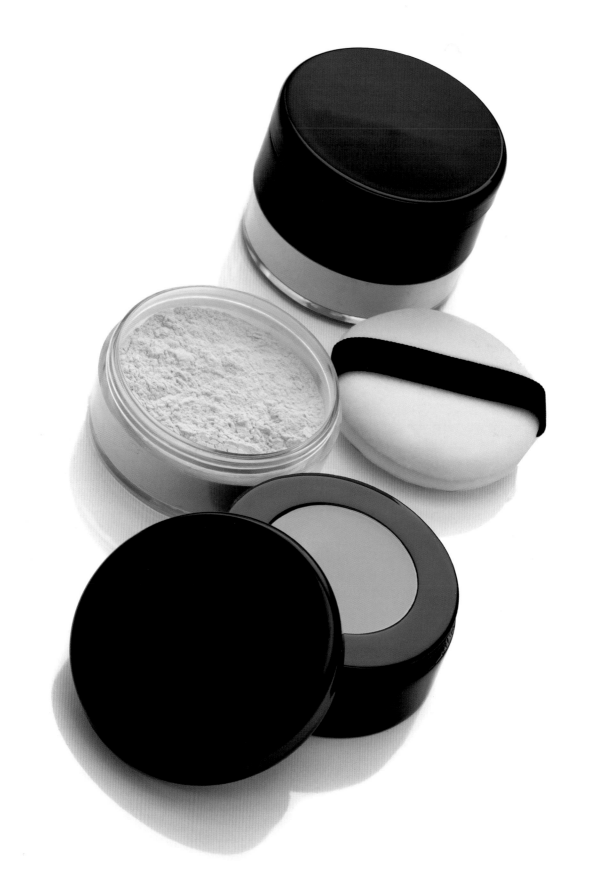

16 CREATING THE PERFECT CANVAS

Before you put a single dab of makeup on your face, there are four things you need to do:

1. Prepare: The first step (and you only have to do this one every six months or so) is to get yourself organized. Clean out, unclutter, and simplify your makeup drawer so that only the products you really love and use are front and center. (See chapter 15 for organizational tips.)

2. Observe: Look at yourself in the mirror and honestly assess how you look this morning and how much makeup you actually need to look your best. (Really don't like what you see? Turn to chapter 24 for bad day beauty tricks.)

3. Decide: What skin care do you need to use to prep your face for makeup? (See chapter 13.)

4. Think: How do you want to look today? Sporty? Polished? Trendy? Sexy? Minimalist? And how many minutes do you have to get ready? (See chapter 19 for time-defined strategies.)

Concealer: The Secret of the Beauty Universe

No matter what, always reach for the concealer first. I don't care if you've only got thirty seconds to get ready, concealer is the one thing you do not skip. Why? Because it's the only way to cover up dark under-eye circles. It works (ideally) by lightening the dark, thinner skin under the eyes to give the illusion that your skin is actually the same color as the rest of your face, making you look less tired.

Bad concealer is, unfortunately, all too common. Good concealer, on the other hand, is the best gift I can give any woman. How do you know the difference? Easy. A bad one is white, pink, chalky, dry, or greasy. It makes you look just plain bad and may even emphasize the very flaws you are trying to cover up. Good concealer is smooth, creamy, and yellow-toned; it blends into your skin easily; and putting it on makes you look instantly better.

The Test. Feel the concealer between your fingers. Does it feel powdery, sticky, thin, or greasy? If so, pass on it. You want one that feels creamy and easy to blend. It should have a yellowish tone. (The exception is if you are truly porcelain white. See chapter 20 for special tips for your coloring.) And it should be just one shade lighter than your skin. Most women pick one that is too light. If you apply the concealer and it looks obvious, chances are you need a slightly darker shade.

Bobbi's Technique for Eliminating Dark Circles

- First, put on a bit of light eye cream (under the eye only) that absorbs quickly into the skin and leaves the under-eye area smooth. If the skin is too dry, the concealer will cake and look crinkly.
- Use a concealer brush (see chapter 14 for brush guidance) or your index finger to apply the concealer in thin layers and blend well. Bring it all the way up to your lash line and into the inner corners of the eyes (making sure you get all the redness, not just the dark circles). This will give your eyes that open, clean look we used to have when we were younger and didn't have such dark under-eye circles. Use more than you think you need and blend it into the skin.

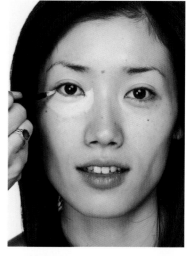

- Don't put any concealer on your eyelids; it'll make your eye makeup crease.
- After applying, use your finger in a soft patting motion to blend it in. Be gentle—you don't want to rub it away!
- Still see dark circles? Apply a second layer of concealer just as you did the first, making sure to pat it in again so that it doesn't crease.
- When you're satisfied with the way it looks, apply foundation to the rest of your face (see page 100 for technique). Next, apply a pale yellow loose powder (or white, if your skin is porcelain), using a soft velour puff, over the concealer and on the eyelids. The powder will lock the concealer in place, make it last longer, and help to further brighten the eye area.

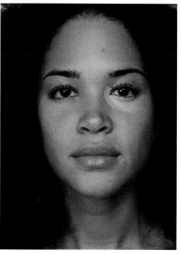

Those are the rules for covering dark circles, and like any rules, there are a few exceptions. If you have reverse circles (lighter than the skin on the rest of your face), you need to experiment with concealer shades. Try one that is the same color as your foundation or a shade darker. If you have very dark, almost purply-green circles (common among some darker skin tones), choose a concealer that's a little bit pink. It would look ashy on most of us, but it works like magic on this problem. Still use a pale yellow powder on top as that will help the concealer blend into the skin tone.

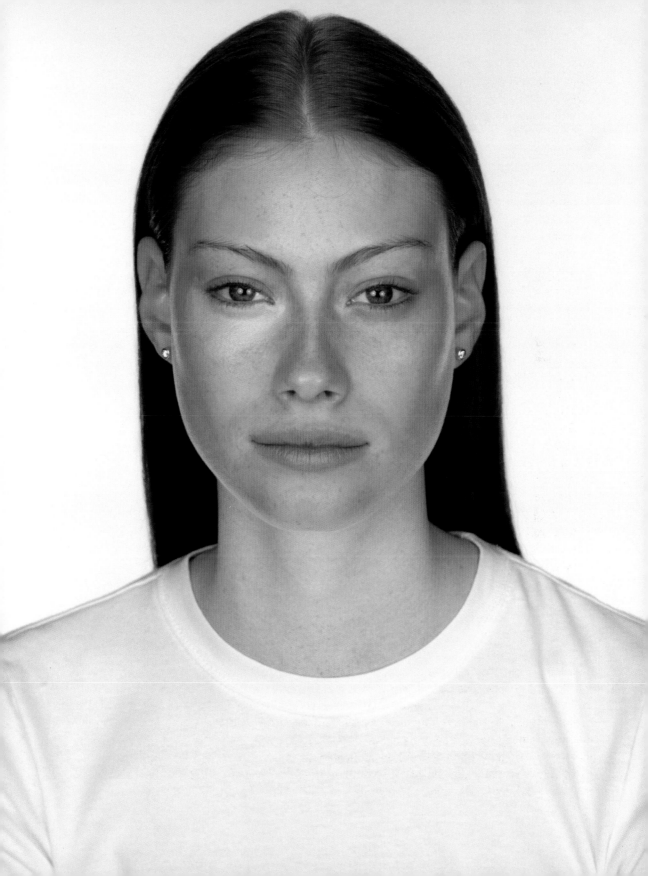

Concealer is not meant for covering blemishes or red spots on your face. Why? Because the right concealer is a shade lighter than skin—use that on top of a blemish and you will actually make it stand out even more. But you can use your concealer to cover up certain birthmarks, sunspots, or age spots. You'll have to experiment a bit, probably using a combination of concealer and foundation in one or two shades. Use a concealer brush to apply product just to the spots you want to cover then finish with foundation (a stick foundation can be ideal for this because it covers and blends easily). Also, do not even try to cover moles. It just doesn't work! You have two choices: Either enjoy them (they worked for Marilyn Monroe and Cindy Crawford) or have a dermatologist remove them. Makeup is not the solution to this problem.

TWENTIES AND THIRTIES CONCEALER TIPS
Even if you don't think you need to wear eye cream, you do need something to moisturize the under-eye area before applying concealer. Without it, the concealer won't go on smoothly. So apply just a dab of eye cream or your regular moisturizer under your eyes before grabbing the concealer.

How to Cover a Blemish

- Apply foundation to your face as usual.
- Then take a concealer brush and dip into a cream or stick foundation (liquid won't give enough on-the-spot coverage) in a shade that matches your face exactly.
- Paint it onto the blemish gently and blend (don't rub) with your finger.
- Take a small amount of powder on a puff and lock it into place.

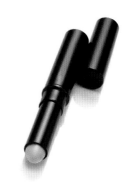

Foundation: The Base of a Great Face

The reason we wear foundation is to even out our skin tone, not to change the color of our skin and not to cover lines (it would have to be so thick and pasty to do that that it would look horrible). Since the goal of a good foundation is to even out the skin tone, the only way to choose one is to match it exactly to the side of your face. You're going to wear it on your face, so matching it to the back of your hand or the inside of your arm (usually a very different tone than your face) is pointless. The idea is to find one that blends into your skin exactly so that when you put it on, it makes your face look smooth and flawless and looks as though you're not wearing foundation at all.

Bobbi's Rules for Choosing the Perfect Foundation

- Take your time choosing the foundation that is right for your skin in both color and texture. The payoff is worth it: Just as the right underwear makes the clothes you put on look better, the right foundation makes the rest of your makeup look perfect.
- Only buy foundation that you can actually test on your face.
- Always check the color in the daylight. Since most stores have

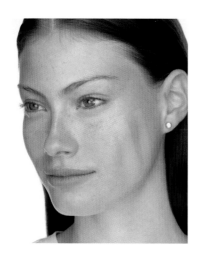

very little natural light, apply the foundation to your face and then go outside with a small mirror to really look at it before you buy. (Turn your face to the side to see if it blends in and matches the color of your neck.)

- A foundation with a yellow tone (not pinkish) is the way to go.
- Make sure the formula is the right one for your skin type.

Since your foundation needs to match your skin exactly, you will probably need to have two different shades—one for the winter months and a slightly darker one for the summer (no matter how careful we are with our sunscreen, our skin color does warm up in the summer). Blend your two shades together during those in-between times when your skin doesn't match either foundation perfectly. Except for extremely fair, porcelain skin tones, everyone really needs a foundation that has a yellowish tone to warm up the skin. And the darker your skin, the more a yellow-toned foundation becomes a must (though many foundations also have a reddish, orange, or blue tone mixed with the yellow that works on dark skin). A pinky beige foundation will look too fake and makeup-y. You'll end up looking like you're wearing a mask, especially in a flash photo.

Once you've found the right color, it's time to think about texture. Choosing the right foundation formula means finding the one that works best with your skin type. But your style and how much makeup you like to wear can also dictate what foundation to choose. I keep more than one type on hand so that I have choices depending on my mood and on the occasion. I use a stick for every day (because it's portable and easy to apply only in the spots where I need it). In the summer or on weekends, I often opt for tinted moisturizer. And when I want more coverage (for a black tie party or a business appearance), I wear a moisturizing cream liquid. Experiment with several until you find what suits you best.

Dry skin. Your choices are stick, cream, liquid, or whipped—all with oil. Make sure the formula you choose doesn't have a powdery feel; never use oil-free foundation because it will make your skin look dehydrated. And cream-to-powder formulas can feel chalky and make skin look even drier.

Normal skin. You can choose any formula you like.

Oily skin. Don't even think of wearing anything except an oil-free formula—whether it's a stick, liquid, or cream. You can further diminish the oil by using an oil-control lotion in your T-zone before applying foundation and using an oil-free powder, applied with a puff, on top of foundation.

Combination skin. You should use an oil-control lotion on the parts that are oily and moisturizer on dry areas, like cheeks, before applying foundation. You may need to switch formulas based on the seasons—oil-free during the summer, a more moisturizing one for the winter months.

Applying foundation so that it looks completely natural should be extremely easy—as long as you've managed to find the right shade of foundation. It should match your face so perfectly that you could even get away with putting it on without a mirror if you had to. I like to apply my foundation directly onto my face (just dot it all over) and then use my fingers or a disposable makeup sponge to blend it in. You can apply it to your entire face or just in spots that need a little coverage or evening out—the trick is just to be sure to blend it in seamlessly. And no, you don't need to apply foundation to your neck—if you are using the right shade of foundation there shouldn't be any line of demarcation between your face (where the foundation is) and your neck (where it isn't).

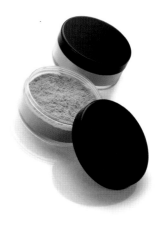

TWENTIES AND THIRTIES POWDER TIPS

Powder is a great way to make oily skin shine-free, but be careful not to be too heavy-handed. Whether you apply your loose powder with a puff or a brush, be sure to use a large brush to sweep off any excess. And keep a compact of pressed powder (that is the right match for your skin tone) on hand to combat midday oiliness.

Powder: Keeping It All in Place

The purpose of powder is to keep foundation on longer, add a little more coverage, and take away shine. A common mistake women make is to think that translucent powder is transparent. It's not. Translucent powder is actually a pale grayish-pink tone that looks totally artificial and can make skin look pasty. I'm a firm believer in the power of warm yellow tones to add warmth and light to the skin. There is almost no one who needs a powder without yellow under-tones. If your skin is so, so, so white (and I've met only one or two women who fit this category), I recommend a white powder, used very sparingly (you don't want to look like a geisha).

Makeup looks very different in the package than it does on your face, so the only way to know if a shade of powder works is to put some on your skin. As with foundation, you will probably need a slightly darker shade for summer, a lighter one for winter. An oil-free, sheer powder is perfect for absorbing excess shine on oily skin. One that contains a bit of oil and feels silky to the touch will be kinder to dry skin (covering smoothly without calling attention to lines). Pressed powder (the kind that comes in a compact) is great for touch-ups during the day. But you should have loose powder at home for when you first do your makeup. I prefer to apply powder with a puff and then use a large brush to wipe off the excess. For oily skin, apply a fair amount. For drier skin, use only around the nose and forehead. And on days when your skin feels really dry, you can go without.

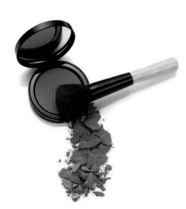

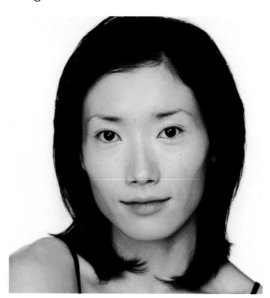

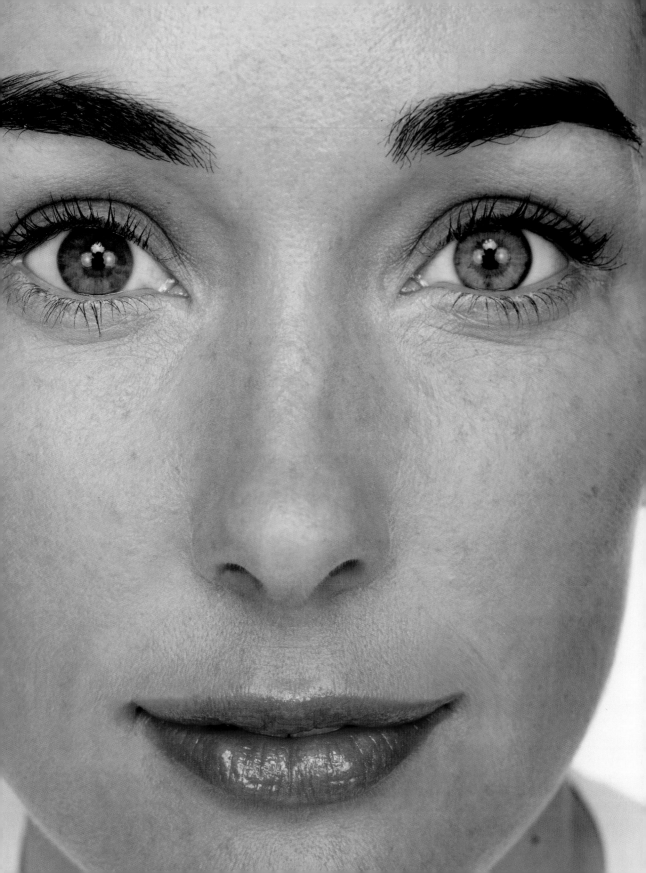

17 **ALL ABOUT EYES**

Eye makeup is designed to make eyes stand out. Wearing eye makeup can backfire, however, if you choose shades that compete with your eye color. The secret of good eye makeup is quite simple: Enhance your eyes. That can mean anything from just using mascara or lining the eyes to wearing a full eye of liner, shadow, contour, and mascara. And while a bold, brightly colored eye shadow can look fabulous in a magazine photograph, real women should stick to more muted neutral shades. Whatever you choose, the goal is to make sure it's your eyes that get noticed—not your eye makeup!

Before you apply any shadow or liner to your eyes, dust your pale yellow face powder onto your lids. This works like a base for your eye shadow to adhere to. And then build from there. Just choose a light color for all over, medium for lid, and dark for eyeliner. Your optional fourth color is to contour between medium and dark ones.

Eye shadow base. Choose a color that blends into your skin tone (especially for day), such as white, bone, toast, sand, or banana. What doesn't work? Pink, rose, or any shadow with a red tone—it will make you look tired. And since the purpose of this shadow is to blend into the skin, apply it with a fat eye shadow brush to get a lot of shadow all over the lid, from the lashes up to the brow bone.

Lid color. This should be a medium-toned shadow that doesn't require blending and that you apply on the lid, up to the crease. Start with a couple of basic neutral shades before experimenting with anything more dramatic:

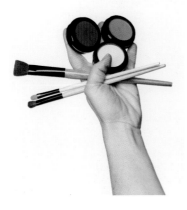

For blue eyes—ashy taupe, gray, heather
For green eyes—yellowy taupe, camel, heather
For brown eyes—rich taupe, sable, mocha

Use a soft, fluffy eye shadow brush and apply the color close to the lashes, over the lid, and three-quarters of the way up the eye. If you have to work too hard to blend it, the color is too dark.

Contouring color. Using a deeper lid color to define the eyes is an optional step for daytime (at night, it's the best way to make eyes look more dramatic). But if you have small eyes, droopy lids, or deep-set eyes, it's worth taking this extra step. Use a medium-wide brush, about the size of a fingernail, either cut on an angle or straight and fluffy. Start at the upper outside corner of the eye and sweep the shadow in and down toward the crease. Sweep a second stroke of shadow, starting at the outside lower corner of the eye at the lash line, and bring it in and up to the crease. Then blend the edges of both lines with your finger. Be careful not to use too dark a shadow; this will only make small eyes appear even smaller. Experiment with color—brown, slate, and mocha all work well. Don't use black or charcoal unless you're going on stage. Smoky black lids are for rock stars and supermodels only!

Liner. This is where you get to use a darker shade—mahogany, charcoal, navy. Bright colors don't work because they will fight with the rest of your eye makeup. You can line just the top lid (be sure to line all the way across—doing it only halfway looks unfinished), but doing just the bottom will make you look tired. To really make eyes stand out, line all the way around the eyes, doing the top lid first. Use a liner brush and apply as close to lashes as possible. Don't worry if it's not perfect; use your finger or a Q-tip to smudge it.

Three Ways to Draw the Line

1. Shadow liner: You apply it with a brush and can use it either dry or damp. This is my favorite because it's very forgiving and easy to blend away if you apply too much.

2. Liquid, cake, or gel liner: This will give you the most dramatic results (good for evening), and it's always applied with a small, thin liner brush. But once it's on, it's hard to fix mistakes without taking it off and starting over.

3. Pencil liners: These are easy to handle, but they don't always have the most staying power. A creamy pencil is great for smudging, but you need to apply a sweep of powder shadow over it to keep it from fading and smearing. Cream-to-powder pencils give a look that's similar to shadow.

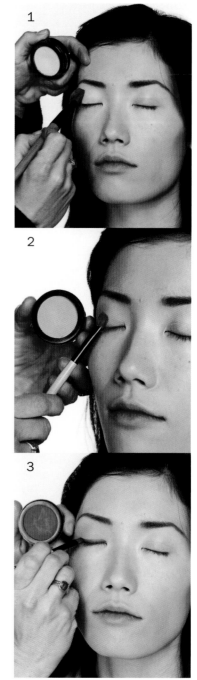

EYE MAKEUP 1, 2, 3:
1. **Light shadow all over.**
2. **Medium shadow on the lid.**
3. **Use a darker shade to line the eyes.**

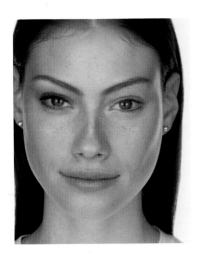

Bobbi's Secrets for Eye Makeup That Lasts

- Beware of moisture! Eye shadow needs a dry surface to adhere to. That means no eye cream on the eyelid—only under the eye as a base for concealer.
- Use pale yellow powder, applied with a puff on top of your concealer and also on the eyelid to take away any moisture.
- Use powder shadow or a water-resistant cream formula for the most staying power.
- Line eyes with damp shadow. Or if you use a pencil liner, apply powder shadow on top of eye.
- Finish with a coat of waterproof mascara.

All About Mascara

My favorite mascara is black. I find that when you wear black mascara, you need less other eye makeup to make your eyes stand out. But women who are especially fair and have light-colored hair and eyelashes should wear brown instead because black will be too harsh a contrast. Color mascara can be fun sometimes and works best with neutral eye shadow. And make sure the mascara is mostly black or brown with color in it—because if it's too bright, it will look too obvious and fake. As for formula, I like lengthening mascara best; it goes on smoothly and makes the most of your lashes without looking unnatural. Thickening formulas often go on clumpy. Waterproof mascara is the right choice for times when you'll be sweating (sports, TV appearances) or crying (like at a wedding, especially your own!). I wouldn't recommend using waterproof mascara every day, however, because it can be harsh and drying to lashes.

To apply: Brush from the base of lashes to tip, applying to the underside of top lashes and the topside on bottom lashes. Apply two to three coats, letting mascara dry before applying the next coat.

To take it off: Apply remover to clean cotton pad and gently wipe over entire eye area. Repeat with a fresh cotton pad until it comes away clean. Follow with a splash of warm water or a damp cotton pad. Waterproof mascara needs its own makeup remover (but the method is the same).

Brows That Wow

Eyebrows are much more important than most women think. The simple step of grooming your brows makes a huge difference in how you look—even if you do nothing else. My advice is to find an eyebrow guru—get a recommendation from a friend—who can groom your brows professionally. Do it once to get your brows into the right shape, and then it's easy to keep it up on your own with tweezing. And anytime you get a bit lazy and your brows become out of control, see the expert again for a fix.

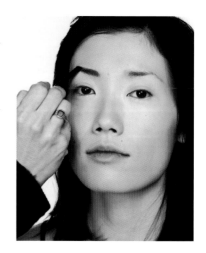

There are several ways to remove hair from your brows—tweezing, waxing, electrolysis, laser—and which you choose is up to you. I personally like the tweezer method because it's quick and gives you the most control. It's worth investing in good tweezers (I like Tweezerman or Rubics) because they not only work better, but they also last forever. I think angled ones are the easiest to maneuver. The best time to tweeze is immediately after you get out of the shower because the pores are open, making it less painful to pull hair out. And of course you need bright light (preferably natural daylight) and a good magnifying mirror. Go slowly, taking just one hair at a time and alternating between brows to keep things even. Don't take too much off without taking a break and stepping back to see how your brows look. You can always go back and pluck more hairs if you haven't taken enough off—but if you pluck too much, you're stuck with skimpy brows until they grow back in.

Bobbi's Step-by-Step Brow Shape-up

- Begin by cleaning up the area in between your brows. Remove stray hairs, but be careful not to take off any hair beyond the inner corner of your eye.
- Brush brows upward (use a brow brush or small toothbrush) and tweeze hairs underneath the brow to create the shape you want.
- If necessary, take off stray hairs above the brows. This is optional, and you need to be careful not to take off too much.
- For brows that are long or unruly, brush them up; then take baby scissors and carefully trim brows. Again, cut only a tiny bit at a time—you can always go back for more.

Even the best-shaped brows sometimes need a little extra definition. Use a brow pencil to fill in sparse areas and powder shadow to add color and definition. How to know what shade to use? That depends on your hair color.

HAIR COLOR	BROW COLOR
Pale blonde	Light ash blonde
Medium to dark blonde	Ash blonde to sable
Light to medium brown	Sable to mahogany
Medium to dark brown	Mahogany to reddish brown

FIFTY+ BROW TIPS

Remember that even though brows fade as you get older, the solution isn't to darken them to the shade they were when you were twenty. The older you are, the lighter your touch should be when applying shadow. Also, check the color in daylight. You want your brows to look natural, not painted on.

Black	Mahogany to smoke (never charcoal or black)
Light red	Taupe or camel
Medium red	Taupe to reddish brown
Dark red	Reddish brown
Slate	Mahogany or dark gray
Light gray	Slate or gray
White	Gray or taupe

Bobbi's Brow-Defining Technique

- Dip your brow brush into your eye shadow powder and tap off the excess.
- Begin at the inner corner of the eye and work your way across the brows with light, feathery strokes.
- Give an extra lift to the eye by stroking some color along the upper edge of the brow to accentuate the arch.
- Check your progress in the mirror to make sure both brows are even. If the color looks too dark or heavy on your face, soften by pressing your yellow-based face powder onto brows with a puff.

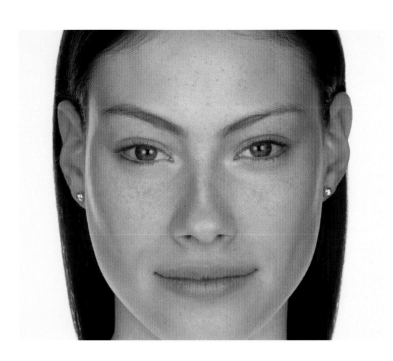

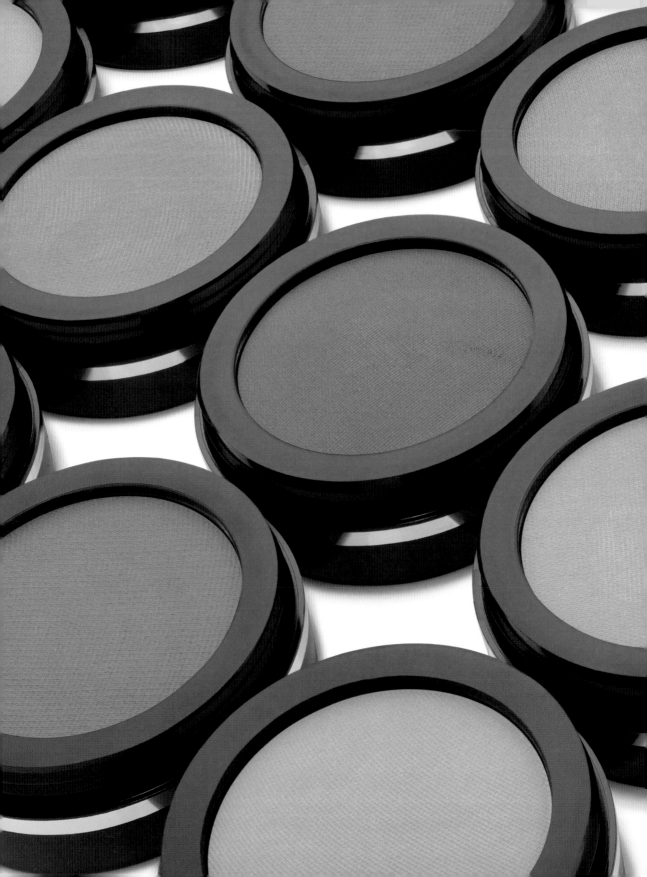

18 JUST ADD COLOR

Do not confuse the concept of natural makeup with a monochromatic, no-makeup look. Makeup that looks natural doesn't have to be all about neutral shades of nude and brown. You need some warm colors on the face to make your skin look alive and pretty. The secret is finding the colors that are just right for your skin.

Blush: A Cheeky Touch of Color

I love blush! After concealer, blush is the cosmetic I can't live without. Putting on blush is the easiest way to look pretty, happy, healthy, and radiant. Many women are afraid of blush because it is easy to get the wrong shade. If you have a shade that fades away an hour after you put it on, or one that's hard to blend into your skin, get rid of it! The right blush is the color your cheeks naturally turn when you exercise or blush. Even if you have very dark or black skin, the right shade of blush gives your face an instant pickup.

Bobbi's Blush Rules

- Find a color that makes you look instantly healthy.
- The right blush should practically blend itself. If you have to work to blend it, the color is too dark or too bright.
- Own two different shades: one that looks totally natural and is the color of naturally flushed cheeks, and one that's a bit brighter for a pop of color.
- In a pinch, use your lipstick on your cheeks as you would cream blush.

The first thing you should do when you bring home a new blush is throw away that little brush that came with it. Those brushes are so skinny that they leave a stripe of blush across your cheek. Choose a larger, fluffier brush instead. (See chapter 14 for brush guidance.) To apply, smile at yourself in the mirror and dab the blush on the apple of cheek, blending up into the hairline. My trick is to also blend down to truly soften the color and make it look like it belongs on your cheeks. Add a pop of a brighter color just on the apple of the cheeks to guarantee that you don't look washed out in an hour. The same basic technique applies to using cream blush: Dot it on the apple of the cheek and use your finger to blend it up to the hairline and down.

A BOBBI SECRET

TAKE YOUR BLUSH FROM DAY TO EVENING BY SWEEPING ON A BRIGHTER SHADE AND BLENDING IT A BIT HIGHER UP ON YOUR CHEEKBONE.

Bobbi's Guide to Just the Right Blush of Color

- **Porcelain skin:** Pale pink or pastel apricot (never use bronzer or brown-toned blush; it will look dirty on your white skin)
- **Fair skin:** Sandy pink tones
- **Medium skin:** Tawny brownish pinks
- **Tan skin:** Deeper brownish rose
- **Latin or light black skin:** Plum, golden brown, or deep rose
- **Black skin:** Dark or deep bronze or deep red
- **Very black skin:** Just a hint of very dark bronzer or no blush at all
- **The second shade:** The extra pop of color—choose anything that's a bit brighter than your regular blush, and one that works well with your lipstick

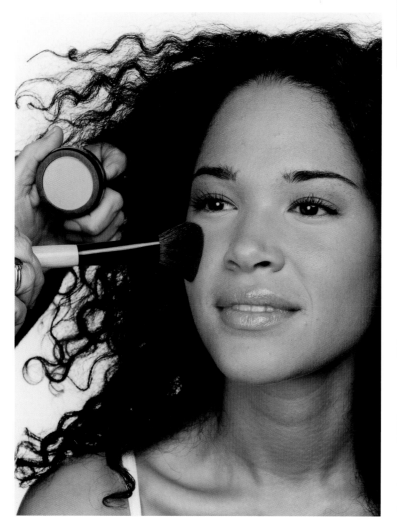

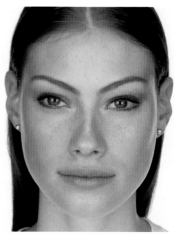

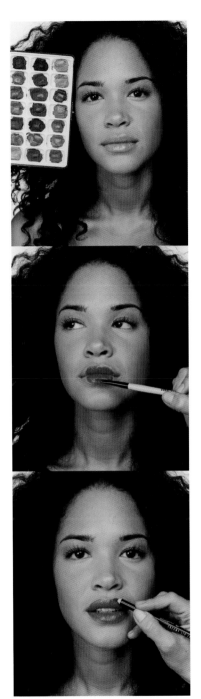

Lips: Color Them Beautiful

Finding the perfect lipstick is at the top of most women's beauty shopping lists. But there is no one perfect lipstick. The best color is going to change—from season to season, by occasion, with age, and with your mood. My advice is to find a couple of great all-the-time colors and then learn how to morph them into other looks for evening or different seasons.

Your quest for that great lipstick should start with a naked face. Yes, I want you to go makeup shopping without a stitch of makeup on (a little concealer is okay). Why? Because you need to choose a lipstick by looking at the true color of your lips. Your natural lip color is important because it's responsible for what a lipstick looks like on you. It also explains why the same shade of lipstick can look completely different on you than it does on your friend.

The trick to finding the right lipstick is to look for a color that is like your natural lip color but taken up a notch. When you find it, you'll know. It will become your tried-and-true shade that looks good when you're just running to the grocery store or the gym (and have little or no other makeup on). But try not to get locked into just one signature shade. Even if you are typically a bright or deep lipstick person, you can also own a great natural color. And if you are a natural lipstick person, you can also own a few brighter shades for evening—or just for fun. Although I'm not a fan of makeup that's complicated to do, you can mix your lipstick colors—it's one way to save a bad purchase. My advice: Own a beige lipstick and a sheer blackberry to help fix mistakes. The beige will tone down a too-bright shade; blackberry will deepen any lipstick and turn it into a great evening color.

Here's a guide to follow according to your lip color:

LIP COLOR	LIPSTICK COLOR
Pale lips	Beige, sandy pinks, white corals, pale pinks
Medium lips	Browns, rose
Dark lips	Raisin
Purple or dark brown lips	Chocolate, blackberry

Pick a Formula

Matte. This is the longest-lasting formula, and it can be a dramatic look in a dark or bright color. But some matte lipsticks can be drying, so look for one that's both matte and moist.

Sheer. This is a good choice for the color-shy because the formula is very forgiving. Even the darkest-looking shades show up as more

Application made easy: Pick a color, use a lip brush to apply, then line around the mouth with a pencil.

of a stain on the lips. Sheer lipsticks aren't generally very long lasting, but because the color isn't too strong, most can be reapplied without a mirror.

Shimmer. This is also a good way to experiment with a stronger color because the shimmer diffuses it. I think shimmers look pretty for evening; just be careful to find a formula that's not too frosty.

Gloss. I love glosses! Putting on a gloss is the fastest way to make lips look fuller, and it's also great for layering over any other kind of lipstick.

Balm. SPFs are essential when you're outdoors. Wear one on its own while exercising, or use with a lip pencil to add color.

Pencil. I don't think you always need to use a lip pencil, but it is a great way to keep lipstick on longer or when you want a more polished look. When I do use pencil, I like one in a nude shade that blends easily into natural lip color. And don't forget to blend the edges, especially when using darker or brighter colors.

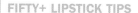

FIFTY+ LIPSTICK TIPS

Your lips will get smaller as you get older—a result of both producing less collagen and your jaw line actually receding with age. Don't try to make them look bigger by drawing outside the lines. Instead, plump them up by wearing softer, creamier (even glossy) shades. To avoid emphasizing fine lines around the mouth, use an emollient, but not greasy, moisturizer on that area.

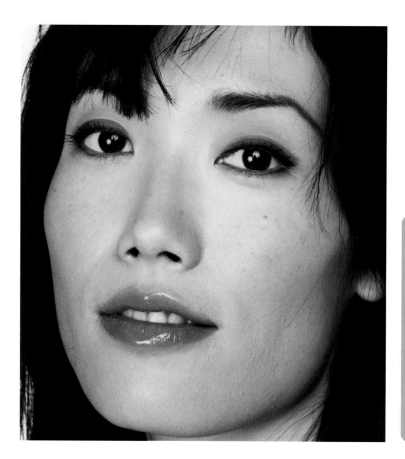

BOBBI SECRETS

YOU CAN PLUMP UP SMALL LIPS BY WEARING A MEDIUM TO LIGHT COLOR. TOO-DARK SHADES WILL MAKE SMALL LIPS LOOK EVEN SMALLER.

GIVE YOUR LIPS EXTRA DEFINITION—AND THE MOST NATURAL LOOK—BY LINING YOUR LIPS *AFTER* YOU APPLY YOUR LIPSTICK.

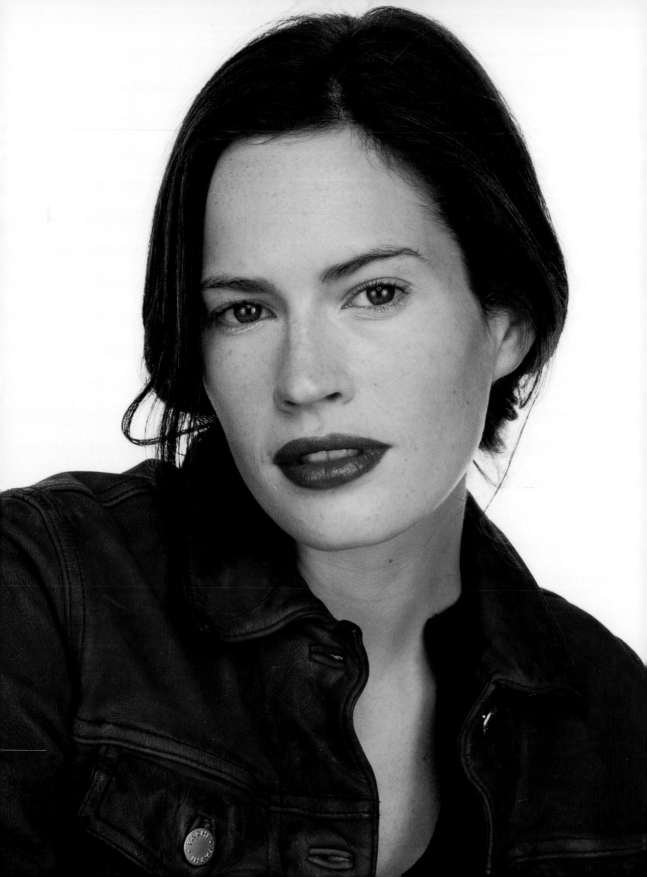

19 TIMING IS EVERYTHING

Five-Minute Makeup

This is the makeup routine to choose when you're truly pressed for time or for those occasions when you don't want to look like you're wearing makeup but don't want to go out with an entirely naked face (running errands, going to the gym, etc.). It's bare bones, but enough to make you look like you didn't just crawl out of bed. I recommend getting an empty makeup palette (a compact divided into several sections) and filling it with your five-minute makeup essentials. In mine, I have a bit of concealer, some stick foundation, cream blush, lip balm, and two lipsticks—a brown and a deeper-colored stain. I can skip eye makeup because my lashes and eyes are dark, but if you are very fair, add a quick coat of brown or black mascara.

Five-Minute Makeup Essentials

- Concealer under the eyes
- Stick foundation around the nose
- Cream blush on the apples of cheeks
- Lip balm with or without lipstick

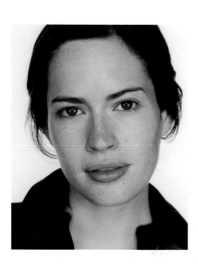
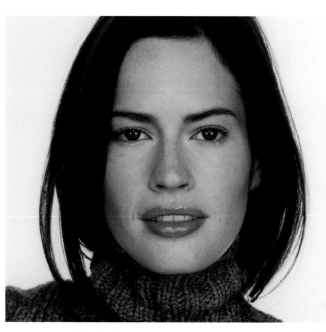

Ten-Minute Makeup

This should be considered your everyday routine—for going to work, going out to lunch, meeting friends to go shopping. It's still fairly quick, but it allows you enough time to put on a full face of makeup. This is the same routine I follow almost anytime I do someone's makeup.

Ten-Minute Makeup Essentials

- Proper skin care (see chapter 13)
- Concealer under eyes
- Foundation blended all over face
- Yellow powder (or white if you have porcelain skin) on top of concealer and over eyelids
- Powder over the rest of your face
- Fill in and shade eyebrows
- Simple eye makeup—light shadow all over lid, medium on lower lid, a dark shade to line eyes, and black mascara
- Blush or bronzer on cheeks
- Lipstick, liner, and gloss
- A spritz of perfume

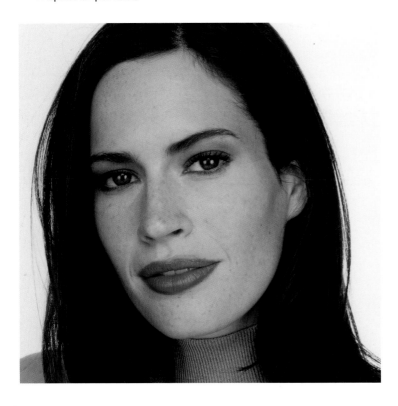

Twenty-Minute Makeup

This is your evening and special-occasion makeup. I don't ever spend more than twenty minutes doing my makeup. If it takes you longer than that, either you are doing too much or your colors aren't right and you're wasting time trying to blend or fix problems. (See chapter 15 for tips on what makeup you might need to toss.)

Twenty-Minute Makeup Essentials

- Same concealer, foundation, and powder as ten-minute makeup routine
- Define brows with shadow and/or pencil
- Try fun eye shadow, such as shimmers or matte shades
- Add a deep medium color in crease of lid to contour
- Black eyeliner shadow, liquid, or gel
- Two coats of black mascara (if you're feeling ambitious, add a couple of individual false lashes on the outer corners of your upper lash line)
- Add some shimmer on cheeks over your regular blush
- Lips can be dark, bright, or pale, but definitely use pencil for more definition and layer gloss on top
- Perfumed body lotion topped with a spritz of fragrance

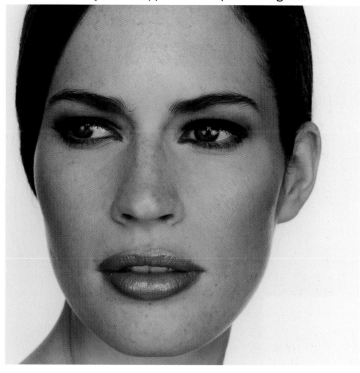

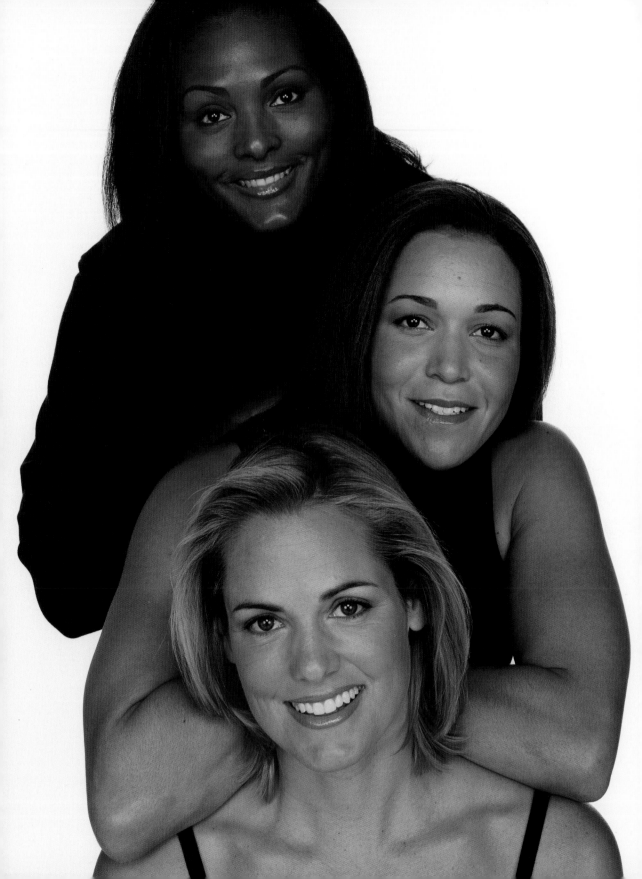

20 BEAUTY BY SKIN TONE

There are makeup tips and beauty rules scattered throughout this book, and the vast majority of them will work for the vast majority of women. But as with any rules, there are several exceptions. Why? Because there is no one face of beauty. There's no one hair or skin color that everyone should try to achieve. And no one ideal of what constitutes the perfect nose, the best color eyes, or the prettiest face shape.

Since beauty comes in such a multicolored, multifaced, and multi-race package today, I've put together some general guidelines to address the biggest beauty concerns I hear from women of different ethnicities. These instructions are for you to use in addition to the tips for choosing foundation and applying makeup found in previous chapters. Follow the ones that work for you, pick and choose rules that suit your own skin tone, and remember that every face, every shade, and every shape has its own unique beauty.

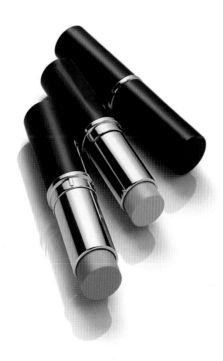

Asian Beauty

I think that Asian women are the most beautiful anywhere in the world. Yet the very attributes I find so stunning—deep-set eyes, wide faces, full lips, and perfectly straight shiny hair—are usually the ones that Asian women complain about. If that's the case for you, my best advice is to appreciate your unique beauty and play it up rather than trying to transform your face into something it's not. For too many years, the models in Asian magazines were mostly Caucasian, and many Asian women are still trying to conform to a Western ideal. That's exactly the opposite of what you should do— you need to accentuate your beauty strengths, not try to imitate someone else's.

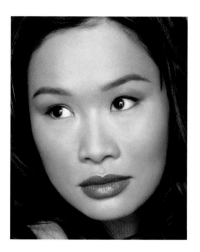

Concealer. Follow the guidelines in chapter 16.

Foundation. Yellow tones are key for Asian women; anything else looks unnatural and masklike. Some Asian women are very fair, others much darker, but all have yellow undertones to their skin.

Eyebrows. Most Asian women have incredibly thick hair on their heads, but very little anywhere else—a bonus when it comes to hair removal, but not always the best thing for eyebrows. The easiest method for filling in sparse brows is to use an eye shadow powder (drawing in extra brows with too much pencil will look fake). I recommend trying a shade like mahogany even if your hair is very dark—never use black or charcoal because it will look too heavy on your face. Dip an eyebrow brush in the powder and then sweep it through brows with light, feathery strokes. If brows are very straight and long, you might want to trim hair a bit and shape them with tweezers to create a slight arch. (See chapter 17 for how-tos.)

Eyes. Don't try to be an illusionist and use eye makeup to create a lid that's not your own. Asian eyes look their most beautiful when they are kept simple. The first rule is to line your eyes all the way around with a deep (not bright) color, making the line much stronger on the top than on the bottom. Make sure it really shows when you open your eyes; this will make eyes stand out. Then take a medium-tone shadow and apply it to the eyelid, sweeping it three-quarters of the way up the lid. The color should be just one tone deeper than your skin tone so that it blends in effortlessly. Using a lighter shade to highlight under the brow bone will help open the eye a bit more. Finish with two to three coats of black thickening mascara to plump up sparse lashes. For evening, smoky eyes look gorgeous, but just

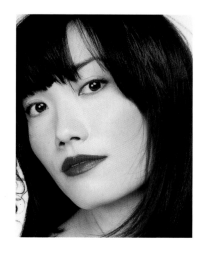

be careful to keep the darkest shadow near the edge of the top lids—sweeping it all over the lid will look too heavy. Shimmery shadow is also a good choice for drawing more attention to eyes because it reflects light and makes the eyes stand out.

Cheeks. Blush is designed to add color, not definition, to the face. Do not try to paint on cheekbones! Just smile and apply a soft pink or rosy blush to the apple of the cheeks to give a hint of color.

Lips. There are no special rules here. Wear what you like. (Consult chapter 18 for color options and application tricks.)

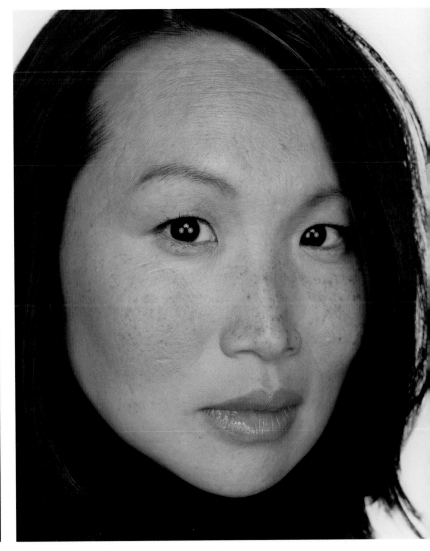

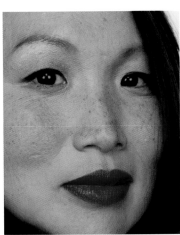

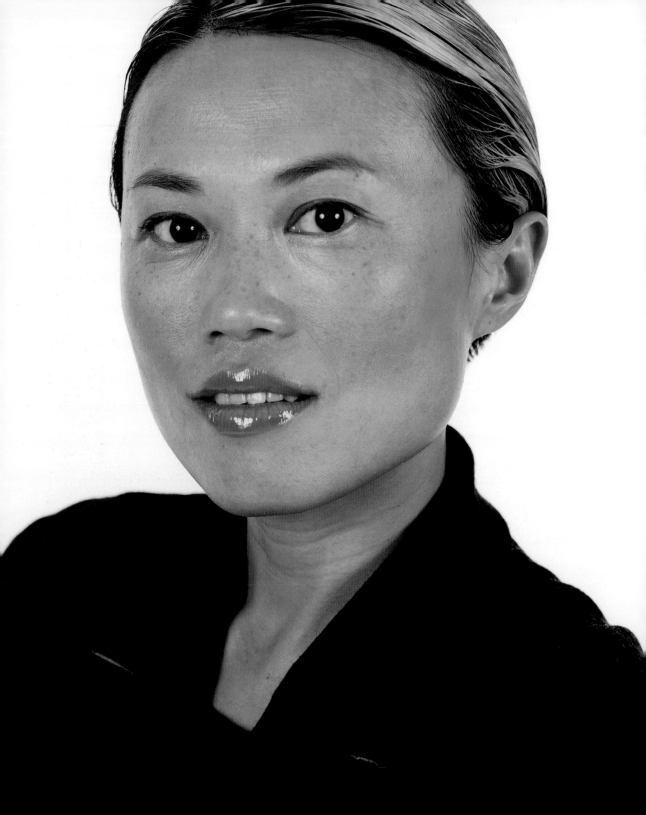

Asian women need to accentuate their beauty
strengths, not try to imitate someone else's.

Middle Eastern Beauty

Women with this coloring exude an exotic beauty that comes from their wonderfully rich skin tone, deep-colored dramatic eyes, and dark, gorgeous hair. But as with anyone, Middle Eastern women also have their share of specific beauty complaints.

Concealer. One of the most common concerns women of this coloring share is very dark under-eye circles. And since your skin tone is unique, the concealer you need has to have very specific characteristics—look for one that has a yellow undertone but with a bit of pink in it to lighten your dark areas. After you apply concealer under the eyes (see chapter 16 for technique tips), seal it in place with a yellow powder both under eyes and on eyelids to lighten the area even more.

Foundation. If your skin has a somewhat greenish tone to it, you need to really experiment with foundation shades. One that isn't an

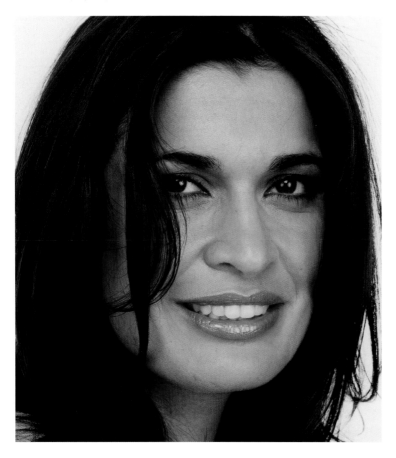

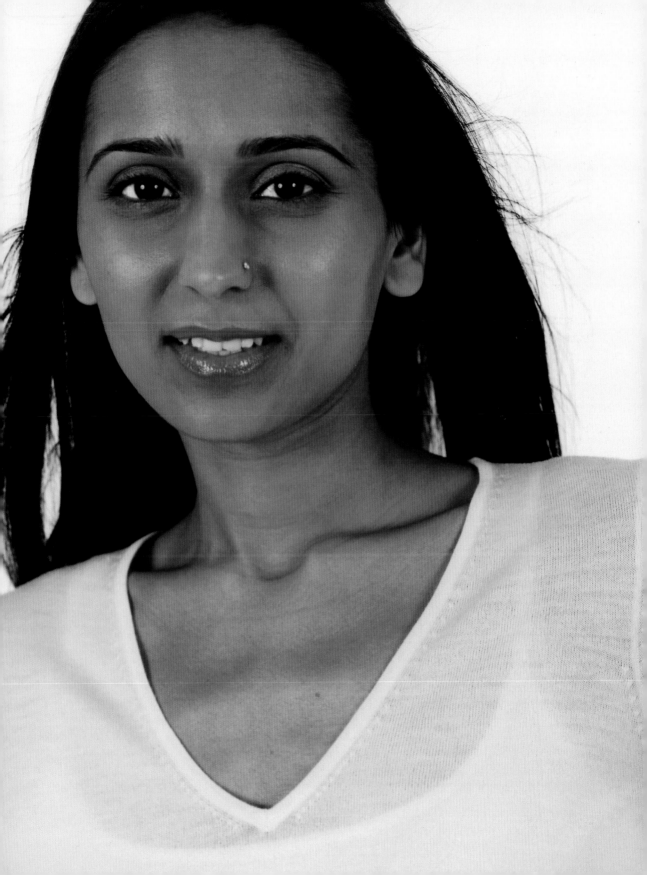

exact match can look pasty and gray on the skin. The wrong foundation will drag your skin down, but the right one—which will have a yellow tone—will smooth skin out and give your skin tone a lift. (See chapter 16 for foundation rules.)

Eyes. For your base lid color, stick to warm tones, such as toast or banana, but not white. You can make a strong statement by lining the eyes with black or smoky charcoal shadow. Using khol to line the inside of the eye may look dramatic, but it will also make eyes look smaller. Then use either golden browns or deep wine shades to add depth. And, of course, black mascara.

Cheeks. Deep bronzer works well as blush, as do plum, currant, and deep rose shades.

Lips. Deep colors look wonderful on darker skin tones, especially on dark blue or black-toned lips. The best shades are chocolate, blackberry, raisin, wine, dark brown, deep rose, and dark red.

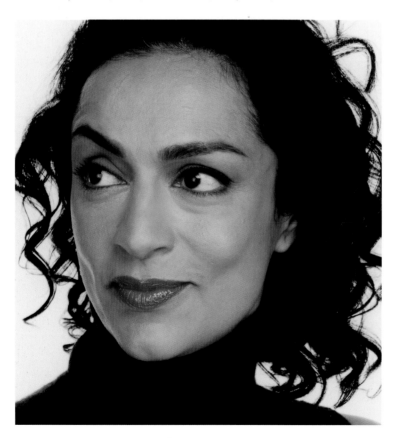

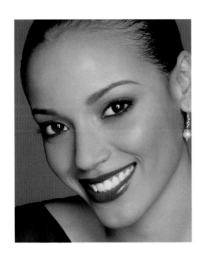

Latin Beauty

When I think of Latin women, I think of women who are seductive and smoldering. I don't know if that comes more from physical appearance or a sexy, self-confident attitude. Use makeup to play up those attributes, and experiment with rich colors and smoky eye makeup. Like all women, Latin women range in coloring from fair and blonde to dark. The one rule that works for all is to make sure your foundation is an exact match to your skin and that makeup colors aren't too bright. Latin women often err on the side of brightness—foundation that's too orange, lips too fuchsia, blush too pink—thinking that those are the best colors to play up their skin. What works much better are natural tones—browns, plums, and deep reds.

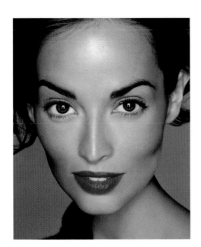

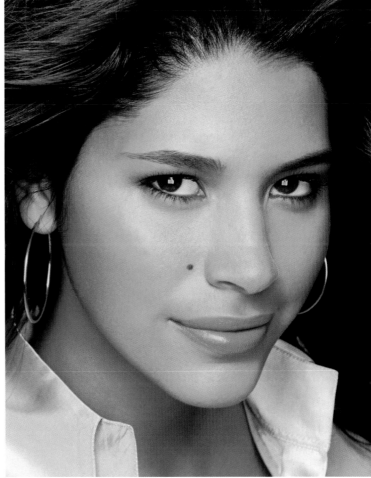

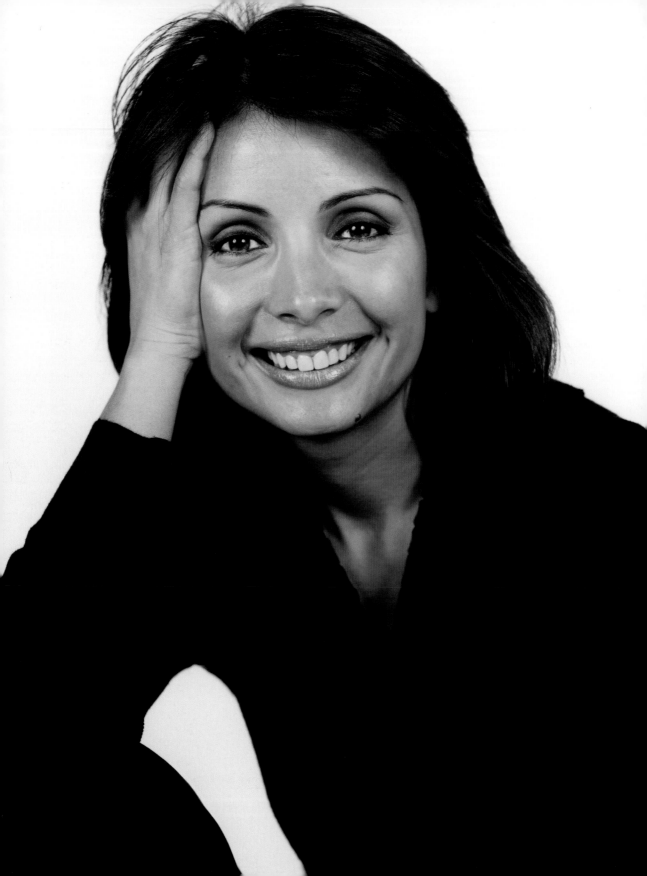

Concealer. Yellow-toned concealer is a must. Follow the guidelines in chapter 16 to find the right shade for your skin.

Foundation. Yellow-toned foundation is the key, but make sure that if skin is dark or suntanned, your foundation has the right golden undertones to blend into your face flawlessly.

Cheeks. Choose soft pale pinks if your skin is light. Go for plums and rose shades if you have a darker skin tone. Stay away from orangey blushes as they are too close to your skin color.

Eyes. Skip shadows that are true purples or blues—they'll look too technicolor on the eyes. My advice is to have two palettes: one of everyday neutrals, like banana, toast, and brown, and another with trendier shades of navy, silver, chocolate, or gold.

Lips. The two big mistakes are too-bright color (like fuchsia) and too-dark lip pencil that's not blended. Try a light lipstick with a dark liner that's blended well into the lips, or a dark lipstick that is sheer enough to let a little of your lips' own color show through.

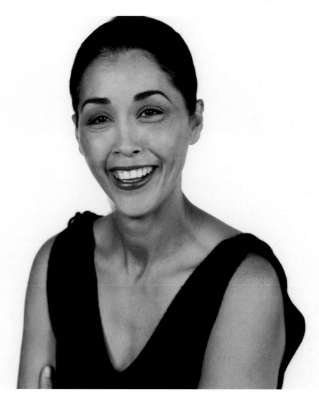

African American Beauty

There are so many variations in skin tones among black women that it can be hard to give general beauty guidance. I know black women who are lighter skinned than I am, others who are a dark mahogany color, and every shade in between. Your skin can be one of your biggest beauty assets, so pay attention to its care. Find what works for your face and body skin to bring out its natural glow. (See chapter 13 for skin care help.) Also realize that some of the features you might see as flaws—like full lips—can become your best feature if you use the right makeup to enhance them. I've always found it ironic (and somewhat sad) that most white women want me to show them how to make their lips fuller and most black women want me to teach them tricks for making theirs appear smaller. The lesson: Appreciate the beauty of what you have!

Concealer. Yellow-toned concealer, topped with yellow powder, will work wonders to lighten dark circles on black skin. (Follow the rules in chapter 16.)

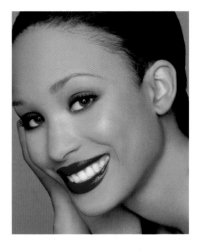

Foundation. Finding the right shade can be tricky for black women, but, thankfully, many makeup companies have broadened their lines to include more options for women of color in recent years. You want to look for a foundation that is yellow-based but with a bit of orange, red, or blue tone, depending on how deep your skin color is. Lighter black skin will need an orange or red tone; very dark skin will work well with a foundation that has a little blue in it. Your skin tone may be a bit uneven—with the forehead and cheeks slightly different shades—so you may need to experiment with using two different foundations on different parts of the face or possibly mixing two shades together for the perfect match. Top with a deep warm shade of powder, which should have yellow undertones. Never wear translucent face powder! It will look extremely pasty and ashen on your skin.

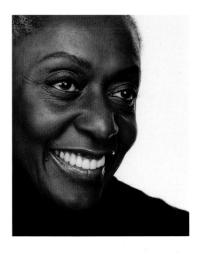

Cheeks. Some very dark black skin looks best with no blush at all or just a hint of very deep bronzer. For dark to medium skin, try a deep bronzing powder or a currant-toned blush. For medium to light skin, plum, rose, or pinks look great.

Eyes. Avoid colors that fight with your skin tone. Lining the eyes with blue or green will bring them out. And on lids, stick with deep, rich shades that blend easily into your skin tone. Chocolate, rich browns, caramel, and toast are great shades to give you a natural

look. Experiment with pale shimmers on the lid, but if they look ashy, skip them and go for more gold and copper shades. Choose a liner color that is darker than your skin to make your eyes stand out.

Lips. The most important advice I can give you about your lips is to love them! Don't try to downplay the fullness because, first of all, it really doesn't work, and second, full lips are incredibly beautiful. There are ways to wear almost any color on your lips—from pale pinks to deep burgundies—and the trick is finding just the right shade to enhance the natural color of your lips. If your bottom lip is paler than your top lip, you can even them out by using a sheer dark lipstick as a base on your lower lip and then applying your regular lipstick to both lips. Or better yet, play up the difference. I think it looks beautiful. I also love the look of light pink lips with dark skin. You can even wear a sheer pink, white, or gold gloss. The secret is outlining the lips with a dark pencil—try raisin or chocolate brown— and blending it really well. You don't want an obvious dark line encircling your mouth. (A good trick: If you can't find a lip pencil dark enough for your skin, use an eye pencil.) If you do choose to downplay your lips, line them just inside your natural lip line.

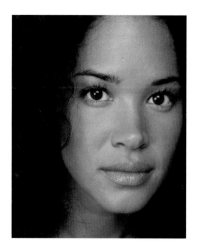

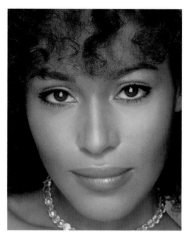

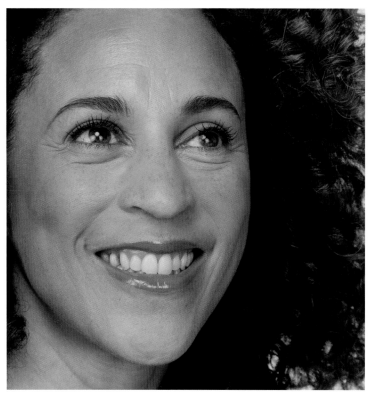

Freckled Beauty

I think that freckles are wonderful. And I hate to see women trying to cover them up. It just doesn't work! So if you have freckles on your face, my advice is to embrace them—because they aren't going to go anywhere.

Concealer. Look for one that is yellow-toned and only one shade lighter than your skin. Make sure it really blends into skin seamlessly.

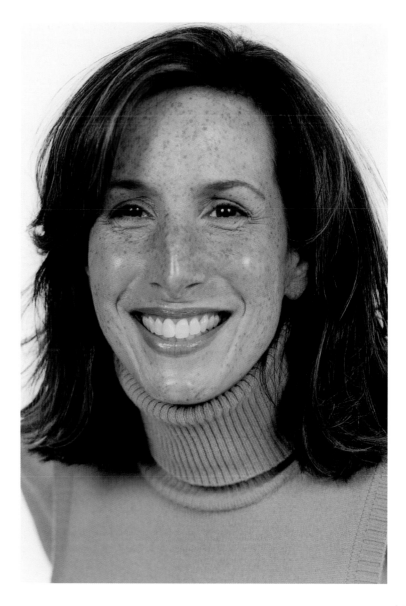

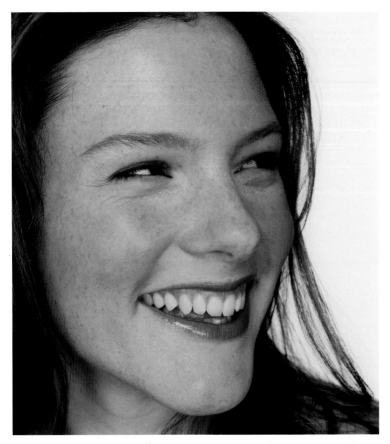

Foundation. Do not even for a minute think of trying to use foundation to cover up your freckles. You'll look like you're wearing cake batter! Most women with freckles don't actually need foundation because their skin tone doesn't need to be evened out. You can use a foundation stick just to spot-cover any redness around your nose or any blemishes. Tinted moisturizer is great on this skin type because it gives some coverage but is sheer enough to let your skin and your freckles show through.

Blush. A light shade of bronzer or sandy pink or tawny blush works best. Avoid plum or hot pink shades.

Eyes. Choose colors that are warm but not ashy. Look for golden tones, yellow, orange, and red-brown.

Lips. Warm reddish-orange shades will look great, or if your lips are pale pink, try a toasted pink shade that has a brown tone to it.

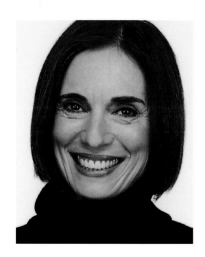

Porcelain Beauty

The secret to making porcelain skin look its prettiest is just letting it be. Don't try to find a self-tanner or bronzer or anything else to warm up your skin. It probably won't work, and you will look much better just staying porcelain. You most likely stay out of the sun, and I'm sure you always wear sunscreen, so you will look younger longer.

Concealer and foundation. You are lucky because you get to use the same color concealer and foundation. A porcelain-colored foundation stick is a good way to cover redness, dark circles, and blemishes. And you are the one skin tone that should not use a yellow-toned powder. Find a white face powder, but use it sparingly.

Blush. Pale pink or apricot blush is the way to go. Avoid anything with a brown undertone—it will make your skin look dirty.

Eyes. Cool tones work best for pale skin; use white, shell, gray, navy, or slate—with black or midnight mascara. Be careful to avoid eye shadows with any red tones in them. They will make you look tired, especially if your skin has any pinkness in the eye area.

Lips. Soft pastel tones, true and clean bright colors, and rich burgundy shades look great. Avoid any lip colors that have brown tones.

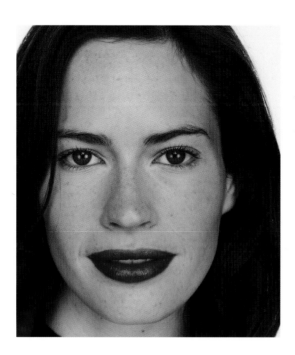

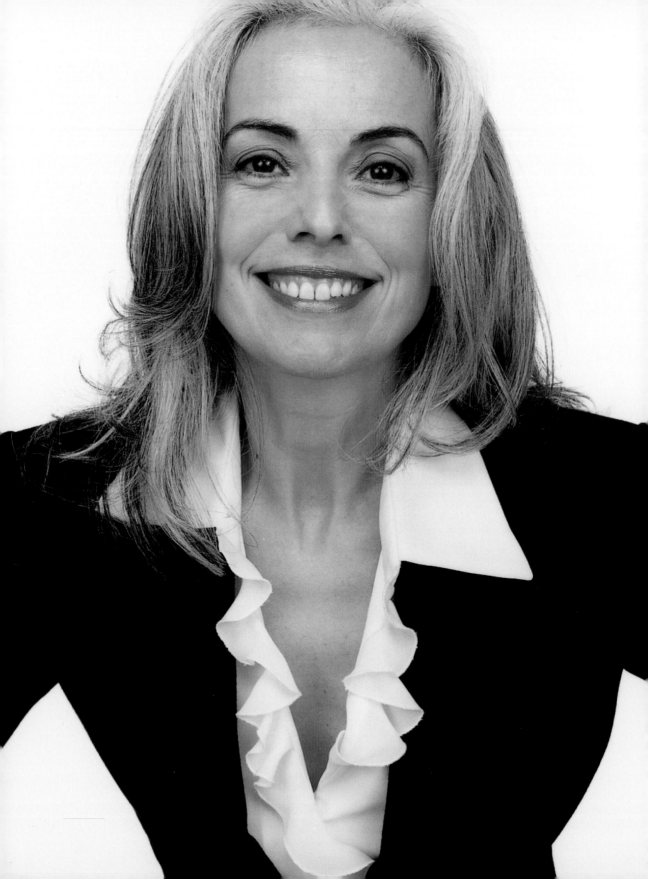

21 BEAUTY BY HAIR COLOR

Does the color of your hair have to dictate the color of your makeup? Not always, but it should play a role. You need to take it all—your hair color, skin tone, the color of your eyes—into consideration when choosing makeup shades. If you still have the same hair color you were born with, you've probably figured out by now which makeup shades compliment you most. The tricky part comes when you suddenly decide to make a radical change in your hair color. If you were a blonde all your life and suddenly decide to become a brunette, the makeup you've always worn will probably look off, likewise for brunettes who go blonde, and for anyone who is newly dealing with gray or white hair.

Even subtle shifts in hair color can have a big impact on your overall look, on the color of clothes that are most flattering, and on the makeup shades that look best. I know for myself that every summer when I have blonde highlights added to my brown hair, I need to switch to slightly more pastel shades than I wear when my hair is dark. The key is just to pay attention to how your hair color (natural or newly acquired) reflects your look.

Usually the first thing you will notice when you change your hair color is that your eyebrows no longer match. Dealing with this is key. Nothing looks worse than a mismatch—like a woman with white-blonde hair and dark brown brows. If you have your hair colored at a salon, ask the colorist to do your brows as well. It's tricky to do on your own, but you can. Just be extremely careful that the dye doesn't get anywhere near your eyes (apply it sparingly to brows), and experiment until you figure out how long you need to leave it on to achieve the correct shade. When in doubt, wash it off sooner. You can always reapply more if brows still aren't exactly the right color.

Even subtle shifts in color can have a big impact.

Ask the Expert

Susanna Romano, owner of Salon AKS in New York City, answers the most common hair color questions:

How do I know if a new hair color will work with my skin tone?
You need to look carefully at your hair color (ideally with the help of a professional colorist) and find a shade that exists in your hair naturally. For example, if you have dark hair that has absolutely no golden tones in it, you will probably look very unnatural if you choose to go blonde. But if your hair has some copper in it, you could color it to a shade in the red or auburn family.

When should I start coloring my hair?
There is no right or wrong answer to this one. Many women look at hair color as just another beauty accessory—and change theirs as often as they might change their lipstick color. Others wait until they have some gray they want to cover, and some women prefer to keep their color real even as it changes over to gray. And while there's no rule that says you must cover those early grays, it does make most women in their thirties and forties (and even fifties) look younger to add a little color to their hair.

What's the upkeep on colored hair?
That will vary tremendously depending on how drastic a change you make. If all you do is a few highlights around the hairline, you can get away with doing it only three or four times a year. But if you go from dark to blonde, that's a serious high-maintenance commitment, and you will have to touch it up about every four weeks.

What are my options if I want to make a noticeable, but not drastic, change to my hair color?
You don't need an entirely new color to make a change. If you want a subtle change—or have just a few scattered gray hairs you want to conceal—I recommend doing highlights that are in the same tone as your hair's base color and maybe two shades lighter. It will bring more light to the face, but it's still very low maintenance.

What's the biggest mistake women make with their hair color, and how can I avoid making it, too?
Too many women overprocess their hair, trying to make it too blonde or change the texture of it. What ends up happening is their hair becomes very dry and loses its shine and elasticity. Taking color out of the hair (which is what bleaching it does) saps the hair

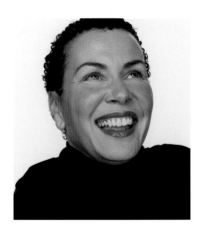

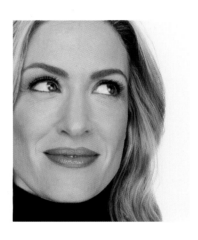

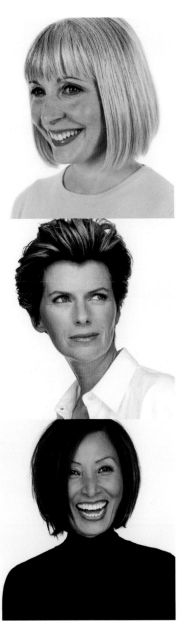

of its natural moisture. So if you are going to go from dark to blonde, you need to be aware that your hair will need extra conditioning and extra care.

Do I need to lighten my hair color as I get older?

Yes, most older women will look too severe with very dark hair, even if that was their natural color when they were younger. That doesn't have to mean going blonde as you get older, but be sure to reevaluate your hair color every so often to make sure it still works with your skin tone, eye color, and eyebrows.

How can I let my colored hair grow in gray—without looking two-toned for months?

There are several ways to ease this transition. First, choose a hairstyle that will help disguise your roots. Cut it shorter, layer it, and wear it without a definite part—that will make the overall effect softer, and your roots less obvious. There are also rinses you can put on your hair that add gloss, not color, and make hair look shinier and the ends a bit lighter. And as more of your gray grows in, you can do reverse highlights—adding a little of your natural color at the hairline. That will make the process less severe and less obvious. The bottom line is, you don't have to go cold turkey on hair color in order to let your hair grow in gray.

I don't want to cover my gray, but I want it to look more vibrant. What can I do?

If you have salt-and-pepper hair, you can get reverse highlights. So instead of lightening the hair around the hairline, you'd darken it. That way you end up with a little more pepper than salt. It looks totally natural and helps your hair not to look too washed out. If you have white hair that is looking a little bit yellow, you need to find a clarifying shampoo that will brighten your white and take the yellow out. And since gray hair can be very dry, it's great to get an occasional deep-conditioning treatment to add back some luster and shine.

Most older women will look too severe with very dark hair, even if that was their natural color.

Makeup Palettes for Every Hair Color

HAIR COLOR	EYES		LIPS		CHEEKS	
BLONDE	BONE	ASH BROWN	SHEER PINK	MEDIUM PINK	SHEER PINK	ROSY PINK
	LIGHT PINK	SMOKY BLACK	BEIGE-Y PINK	SOFT NEUTRAL	BROWNISH PINK	CLEAR PEACH
BRUNETTE	BONE	MEDIUM BROWN	PINKISH BROWN	PLUM BROWN	ROSY PINK	BROWNISH PINK
	MOCHA	MAHOGANY	SHEER RED	SOFT NEUTRAL	ROSY BROWN	SHEER PINK
RED	BONE	MOSSY GREEN	LIGHT PEACH	SHEER LIGHT BROWN	MEDIUM BROWN	ROSY BROWN
	TAUPE	RED BROWN	BROWNISH PINK	MEDIUM CHOCOLATE BROWN	LIGHT ORANGE-Y BROWN	APRICOT
GRAY OR WHITE	WHITE	SLATE	PALE PINK	CORAL	ROSY PINK	CLEAR PEACH
	GREY	NAVY	BRIGHT PINK	MEDIUM PINK	BROWNISH PINK	SHEER PINK

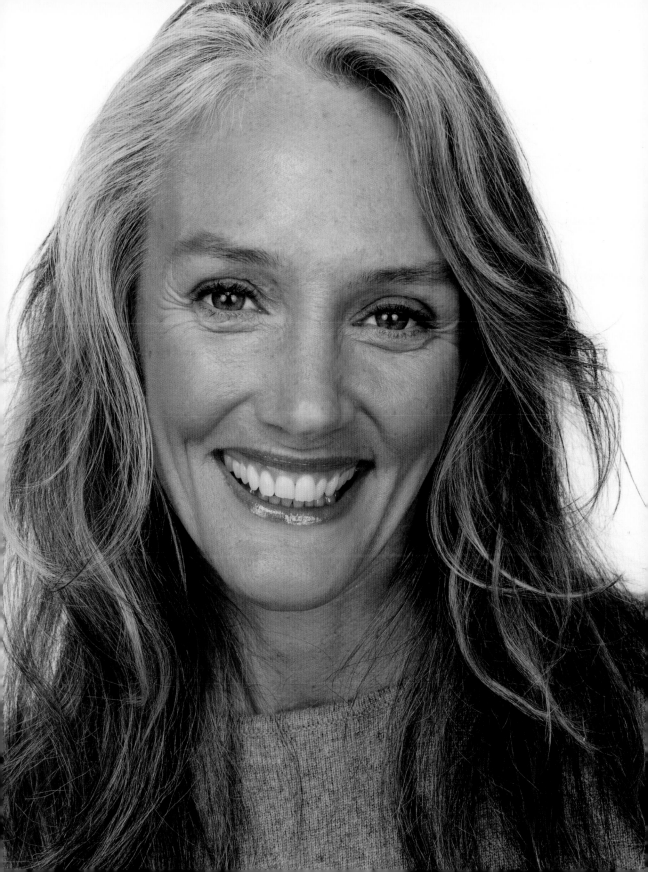

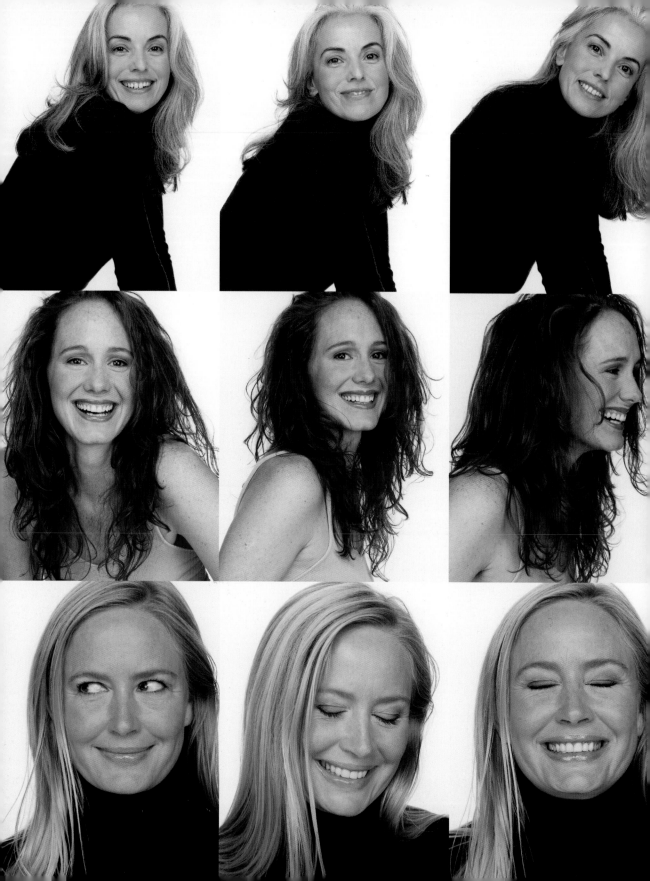

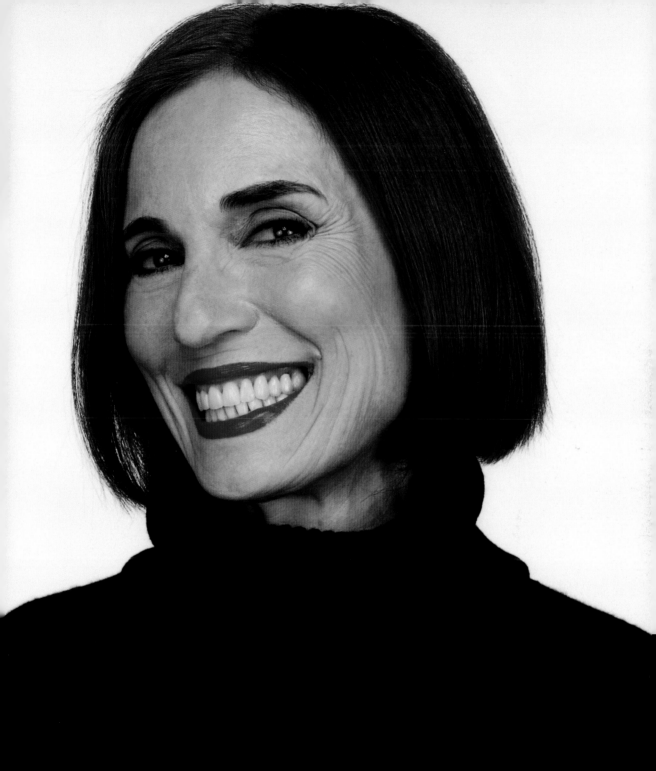

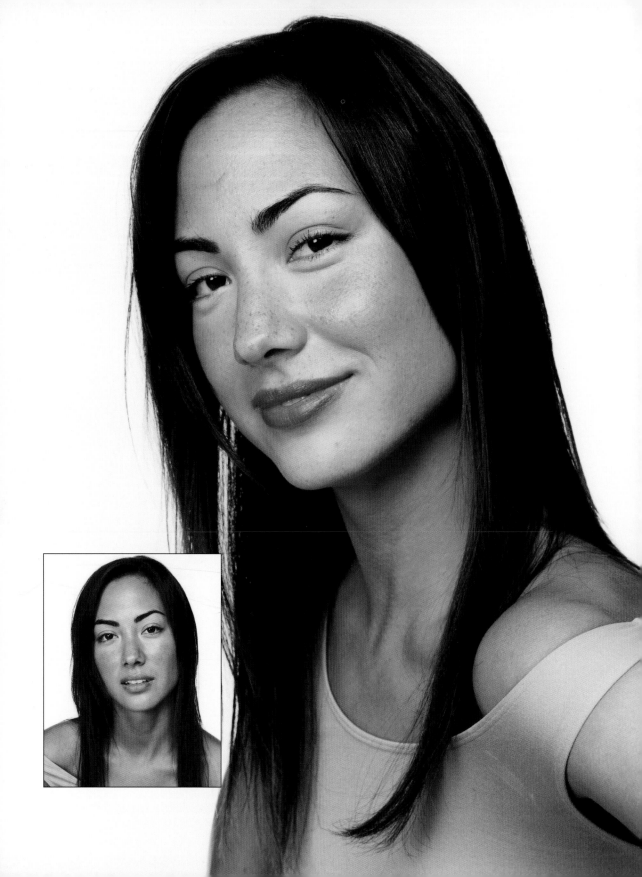

22 MAKE ME OVER

To me, a makeover doesn't have to mean drastic change. Women are always surprised to see that sometimes a major transformation comes from just a few simple adjustments—the right concealer, a few highlights in the hair, or a more flattering shade of lipstick. As we get older, it's easy to get stuck in a rut. And no matter how good that haircut or makeup looked fifteen years ago, chances are it's time for an update. So talk to your hairdresser about a new cut or color, and visit the makeup counter to try a few different shades than what you've been wearing forever. You'll be amazed at how uplifting even a little change can be.

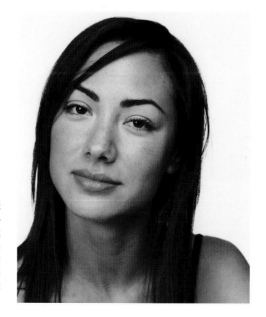

Our model looks gorgeous to start (inset; with just concealer and foundation), but rosy blush and soft pink lipstick instantly freshen up her face and give her skin a luminously healthy glow (big photo). For night, feel free to play with bold color (photo, right), but limit it to one spot only!

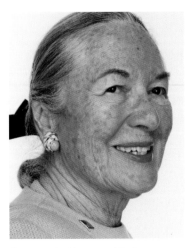

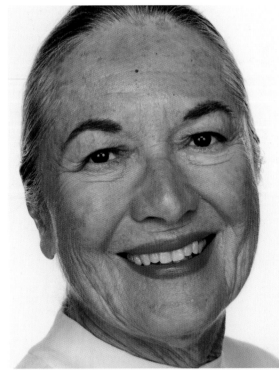

As we get older, our skin tone sometimes gets more uneven. To create the illusion of smooth skin, I used concealer under Jeane's eyes and then a very sheer foundation on the rest of the face—just enough to even out tone. I also defined and darkened her brows and toned down her bright lipstick to a warmer, rosier shade.

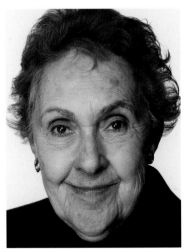

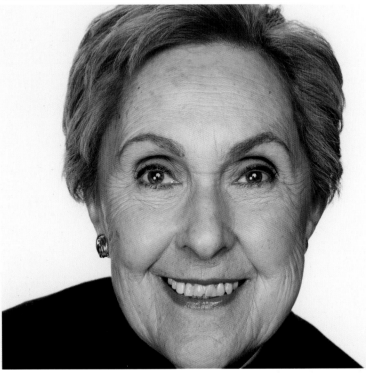

This makeover on Evelyn (my mother-in-law) is a perfect example of what a difference the basics can make. By trimming her hair, adding a few highlights, and blowdrying it straight, her whole face looks lifted. Then just using a pretty blush, glossy lipstick, and defining the brows completed the transformation.

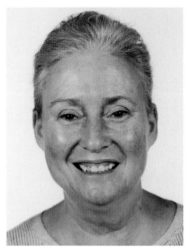

Ruth hadn't changed her look in nearly two decades, and we decided that it was time for her to lose the ponytail. Cutting her hair was a big change, and a change like that usually calls for new makeup. Since the cut brings attention to her eyes, I defined her brows, sweeping neutral shadow along the lids, and adding a darker shade to line the top and bottom lids.

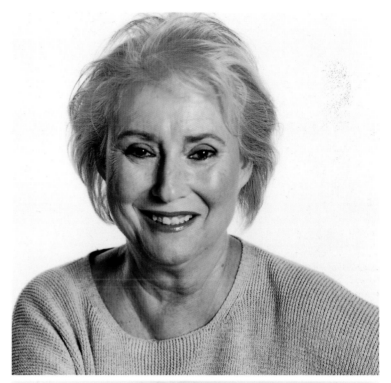

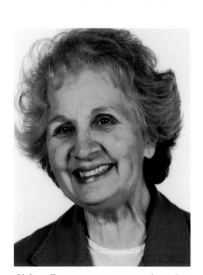

Giving Frances a more modern (no rollers required!) haircut instantly updated her look. And while bright colors can look good at any age, be careful not to go too bold—toning down her fuchsia lipstick to a warm rosy shade is more flattering to her face.

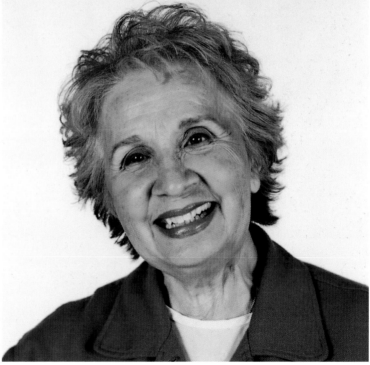

149

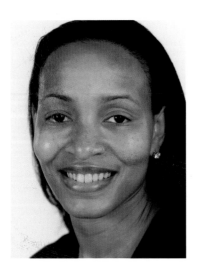

Gina looks absolutely gorgeous completely bare faced, but by smoothing on just a light touch of natural make-up (concealer and foundation to even out skin tone), her look becomes instantly more polished. Below, I took the color up a notch for evening—adding some shimmery, smoky color to the eyes and glossy lips.

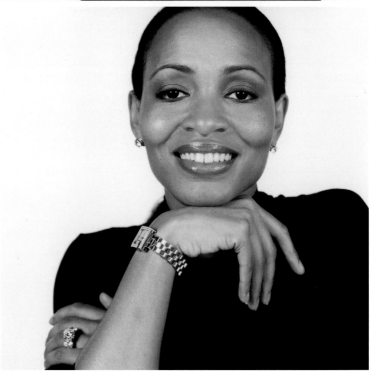

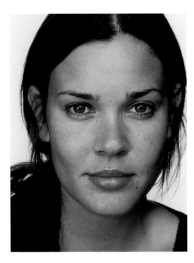

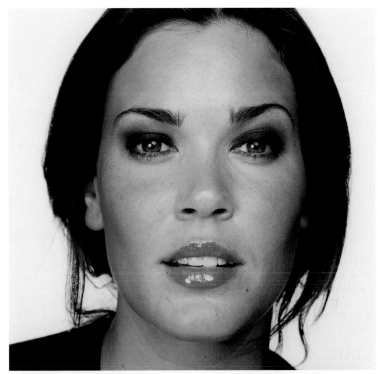

Anna is beautiful without anything on her face (she *is* a model!). But for evening, even the prettiest faces look more luminous with the right shades of make-up. I used a golden-toned foundation to even out her skin, brushed on natural, pink-toned blush and a smoky eye.

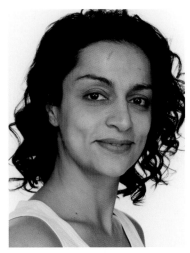

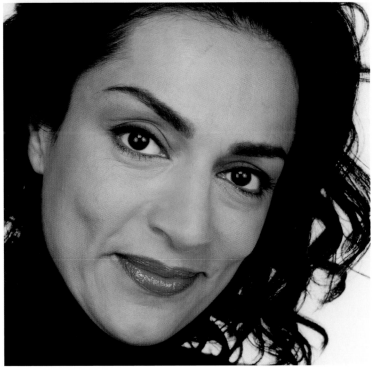

On Ranjana, I used a yellow-toned concealer that has a hint of pink in it to get rid of the greenish under-eye circles. Golden-yellow foundation warmed up her skin and got rid of any ashy undertones. Bronzer works well as blush on darker skin—adding a warm flush of color—and I defined the eyes with a little smoky liner.

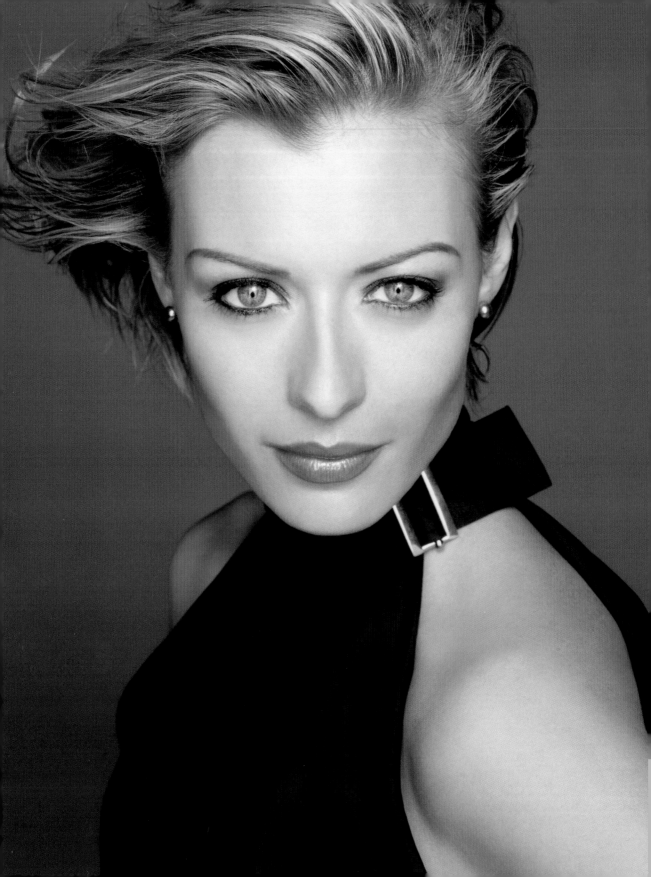

23 MAKING UP FOR ANYTHING

I'm not suggesting that you need to put on a totally different face for every different event in your life, but certain occasions do call for more or less makeup than you normally wear. You always want to look like yourself, but that self will take on a slightly different style, depending on whether you're on a job interview, at a wedding, or on the golf course.

Job Interview

First impressions count, so keep it simple. A lot of young women make the mistake of going on a job interview wearing either no makeup (thinking it'll make them look more serious) or too much makeup (thinking it'll make them look more sophisticated). The ideal look is somewhere in between. You don't want the person interviewing you to be more focused on your fuchsia lipstick than on your resume or your words. The best advice I can give you is that less is better. Your makeup should not be competing with you for

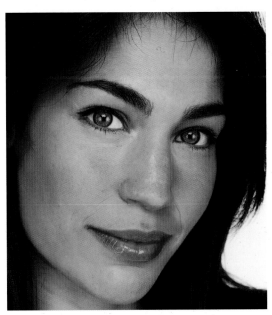

attention. That means sticking with everyday neutrals, nothing too bright, nothing shimmery, nothing overdone. And make certain that nails are clean, with subtle polish that's not chipped. When you arrive at the interview, be sure to take a minute to compose yourself: Go to the restroom, freshen your lipstick, make sure everything is blended, take a deep breath, and relax.

Interview Tip Sheet

- Keep skin simple, which means not too much foundation, just enough to cover blemishes and redness and to even out the skin tone.
- Skip harsh, bright, or shimmery eye shadows. Stick with neutral colors on your lids, such as taupe, gray, blonde, or toast. And save the black eyeliner for evening; an interview face calls for something more natural, like brown liner.
- Choose your style depending on where you are going to interview.

Conservative (law firm, finance, corporate). Keep your clothing classic and simple. For makeup, you need it to look polished and professional, but not overdone. Use foundation and concealer, eyeliner, blush, and a neutral lip color. Hair needs to be neat, whether you leave it down or pull it back. The style shouldn't look overly trendy, and hair shouldn't be loaded down with lots of obvious styling gel or hairspray.

Creative (fashion, beauty, graphic arts, retail). You'll want to look simple, but definitely stylish. Let your own taste and style dictate what you wear; you want to look current, but not like a fashion victim. Your choice of makeup colors can be a little more adventurous, but remember, this isn't a cocktail party. Save the smoky eyes and sparkly powders for evening.

Business casual (teaching, tech companies, nonprofits). This doesn't mean you should wear jeans and a T-shirt. Make sure your clothes are neat, clean, and tailored. You won't want to wear a lot of makeup, but don't go naked. Use a foundation stick to cover blemishes and even out skin, and add a sweep of warm blush and some neutral lipstick.

Night Out

For evening, turn the intensity up a notch. The perfect evening makeup makes you look like yourself, only more gorgeous. Lighting is softer at night, so you want to compensate by doing your makeup a bit stronger and a bit brighter; otherwise you'll look washed out. One of my favorite evening looks of all time was Carolyn Bessette

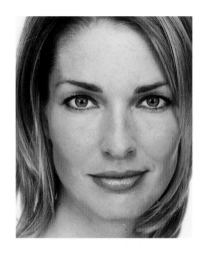

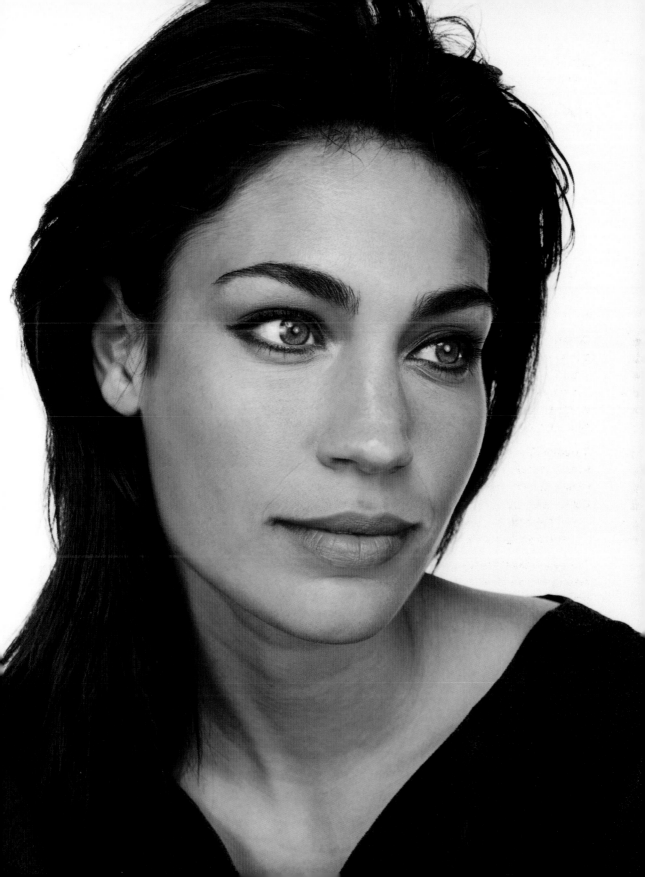

Kennedy's. She would keep her face and her hair very simple and just put on a dramatic stain of red lipstick. Of course, not everyone can carry that off, but everyone can follow that same guideline: Pick one feature to play up and keep the makeup on the rest of the face clean and pretty. Make sure you have enough foundation and blush on to give your face life. Use your everyday foundation, but choose a blush that's a touch brighter than normal. And then decide if you want to play up your eyes or your mouth. Don't do both. If you want a stronger eye, do a softer mouth. Or subtle color on your eyes with a bold mouth. Personally, I prefer doing more with the eyes and less with the lips. It looks beautiful and it's not too high maintenance. When your lips are very bright or very dark, the color will come off every time you take a drink. So instead of running to the bathroom to redo it every ten minutes, I'd rather do my makeup so that it looks great even if my lipstick fades away. (See chapter 17 for eye makeup application tricks.)

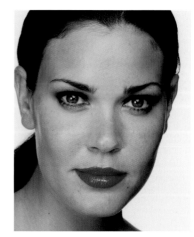

Evening Tip Sheet

- Always brighten eyes with concealer.
- Adding a bit of shimmer (to eyes or lips) is a fast way to make your nighttime makeup special.
- Make lips look dramatic by choosing a shade that's slightly richer than what you'd normally wear for day. If you like berry gloss by day, take it up a notch by trying a slightly deeper burgundy for night.
- Don't ignore your skin. If your neck and chest are bare, sweep on a light touch of bronzing powder, working downward from your chin.
- Make cheeks glow by using a cream blush topped with just a pop of powder blush to the apples of the cheeks. Or try a shimmery blush to add sparkle to cheeks.
- Finish with two coats of very black mascara.
- Switch from your light daytime scent to a warm, sexy fragrance.

Exercise

Active makeup means very little makeup. When you're exercising, even the littlest bit of makeup can look like a lot. If you're going to be outside, the most important thing you need is sunscreen. My absolute favorite sunscreen is BullFrog. It's totally waterproof and nongreasy, and it really helps you not to burn. I also love Banana Boat. (Neither of these is great under makeup, however, so save them for the beach or an outdoor workout.) If you're doing something really physical and sweaty, you don't need any makeup over your sunscreen. But if you're doing something like playing golf—and still want to look polished and pretty when you stop for lunch at the

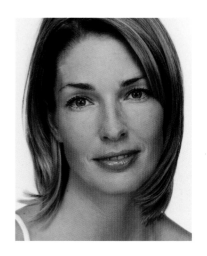

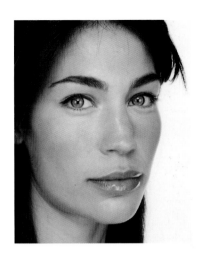

clubhouse—then you can go with a bit more. Try a tinted moisturizer with SPF instead of foundation because it's lighter and looks more natural. Then add a light lip color with SPF, some blush or bronzer, and a coat of waterproof mascara. For cold weather activity, such as skiing, you need even less. But you do need lots of protection for your skin. People often assume that if it's not summer and they're not lying on a beach, they don't need sunscreen. Not true! If you are at a high elevation, even when it's overcast, you get a lot of sun on your face. Use a really intensive moisturizer with SPF 30 or more in it. And keep a small stick foundation in your pocket. Just a touch under your eyes or wherever you need it will make you feel much better when you come off the slopes and head into the lodge at the end of the day.

Photos

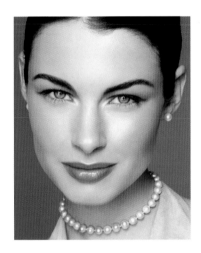

Looking pretty in a picture. A common mistake women make is piling on extra makeup for a photo without really stopping to analyze what they're doing. If you're getting your picture taken, the first thing you should do is think about what the picture is for—whether it's your daughter's wedding, your passport picture, or a corporate press kit—and how you want to appear when you see that photo year after year. Even if I'm just getting my picture done for my license or my gym ID card, I'll do three things: concealer, blush, and lip gloss. Do just that, and I guarantee you'll be much happier pulling that photo out of your wallet every day.

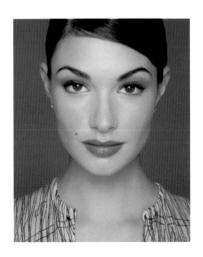

Lighting plays a big part in making you look either fabulous or dreadful in a photo. And you need to take the lighting into consideration when you put your makeup on. If your photos are being done outdoors, try to avoid scheduling them for midday. Midday light is the worst because it causes shadows on the face that play up dark circles and any other imperfections. The most flattering time of day is late afternoon, around 5 P.M. when the sun starts going down. Everyone looks amazing in that soft light. For outdoor photographs, you definitely need some makeup, but don't overdo it. In natural light, a little makeup can look like a lot. For indoor photography, you have to factor in the flash. A flash tends to emphasize pink tones, so be sure to use only yellow-based foundation and powder. And avoid foundations that contain titanium dioxide (a common sun-blocking ingredient)—they tend to be pasty, which looks ashy on the skin, plus the titanium dioxide reflects light in photos.

157

Photo Tip Sheet

- Don't overmoisturize. A dewy complexion (which I normally love) just looks greasy in photographs. Be especially careful of oiliness on the T-zone—forehead, nose, and chin. To prevent this, use an oil-control lotion under your foundation.
- Avoid overfrosted formulas of lipstick or too-shimmery eye shadow—they reflect light and will appear shiny in photographs.
- Define lips and eyes carefully, but avoid super-dark shades. Instead go just one shade deeper than your everyday lipstick. For example, add a deeper color gloss or mix in a deeper pencil in the same tone as your lipstick.
- Black shadow—even as eyeliner—is too dark for most daytime photos. Instead, choose a deep-colored eyeliner, such as mahogany or navy. You can still get away with a smoky eye, but it needs to be slightly less dramatic. Layer two to three shadows in varying shades of the same tone, but keep it close to the lashes.

Weddings

What to do before you say "I do." Wedding makeup should be special, but it shouldn't be a disguise. On your wedding day you want to look like you, but you at your most radiant and beautiful. Like good evening makeup, the makeup you wear on your wedding day should be like your normal makeup, just taken up a notch. Think slightly brighter and rosier lip color, a pretty shade of blush that gives your skin a healthy flush (pink if you're fair, plum if you're dark-skinned), and well-defined eyes. This is not the occasion to try anything too trendy; when you look at your wedding album in the years to come, you want to look timeless, not dated.

Wedding Tip Sheet

- Do a trial run with your makeup before the big day. If anything doesn't look perfect, you'll have plenty of time to make adjustments or buy new shades.
- Think about ways to make your makeup last throughout the wedding—set foundation with loose powder, wear waterproof mascara, line and fill in lips with lip pencil.
- Define your eyes, but use soft colors like bone or white to highlight eyes and a medium charcoal or navy shade to line lids.
- Keep these essentials handy for touch-ups during the reception: concealer, sheer pressed powder, lipstick, lip pencil, and lip gloss.

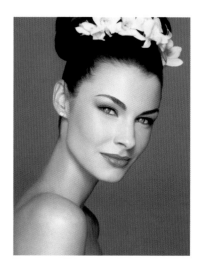

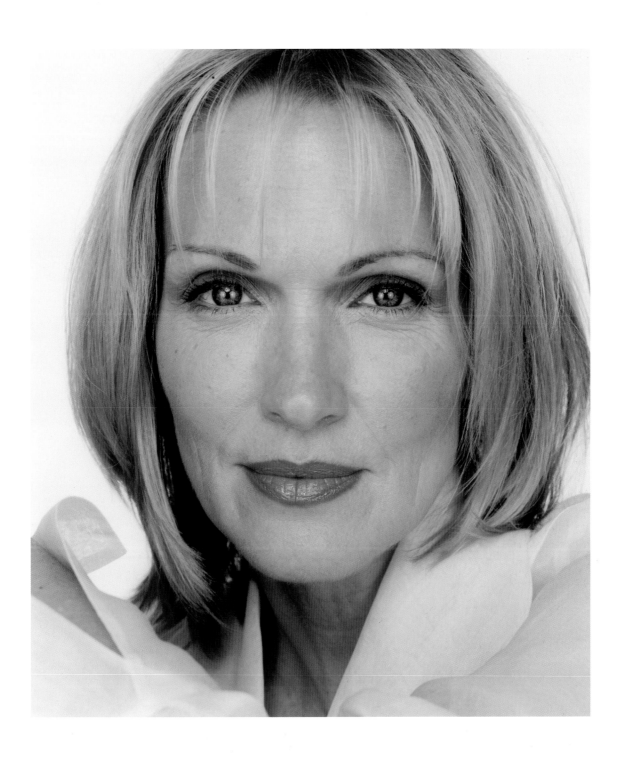

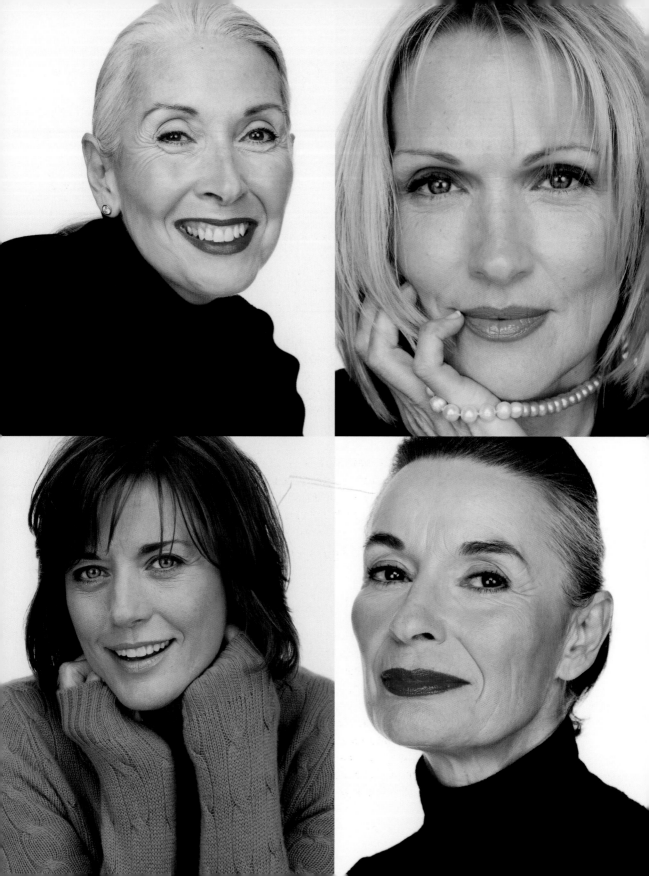

24 BEAUTY EMERGENCY:
QUICK FIXES FOR BAD DAYS

My favorite quote about beauty is: "The best cosmetic for beauty is happiness." So true. But let's face it, there are those days when, happy or not, you wake up not looking your best. Here are a few of my favorite tricks for adding a little more beauty to a bad day.

Wear pink pearls. There is something about the luster of pearls that just makes skin more luminous. And pearls that have a pink cast to them are even better.

Put on some color. For me it's French blue. I always get the most compliments when I wear something that color. Knowing what color works for you is so important. I guarantee you will get compliments when you wear color. And when in doubt, put on pink. It reflects onto your face and automatically makes your skin look fresher and prettier.

Opt for basic black. I know I just said to wear color, but there are some days when you feel so bad you'd rather blend in than stand out. Or maybe you feel a little bloated and know you'll feel thinner in your trusty black pants.

My favorite tricks for adding a little more beauty to a bad day.

Experiment with jewelry. The right jewelry is great because it takes attention away from your face. A great pair of earrings can be the perfect accessory (and distraction) when you don't have time to put makeup on.

Have your teeth whitened. This can make a huge difference in the way you look, literally brightening up your entire face. There are many options for whitening your teeth. You can get custom trays made at your dentist and do the bleaching at home over the course of a few nights. Laser is an expensive, but quick and effective, option. You can get it done on your lunch hour for a big jolt of instant freshness. Both methods can temporarily leave teeth a little sensitive, and neither lasts forever (especially if you drink tea, coffee, or red wine), but I still think it's worth it.

Put on a hat. I don't mean just plopping a baseball cap on your head—although that has saved me numerous times when nothing was going to help. But a stylish hat is an excellent way to hide bad hair and can even make you look incredibly chic the instant you put it on.

Get a new hair color. Whether you choose something as drastic as going from brunette to blonde, decide to cover your gray, or just add a few highlights, having color in your hair gives your face an instant boost. (Just be sure to change your makeup accordingly; see chapter 21 for tips.)

Pull up a ponytail. If your hair is long enough to pull into even the tiniest tail, try it when you're having a bad beauty day. Not only does it mean you no longer have to worry about trying to make your hair look better, but pulling your hair back can work like a mini-facelift.

Fake a tan. If your skin looks a little gray some mornings, faking a sunny glow is the fastest wake-up call. Powdered bronzer is the easiest and most forgiving method for adding some life to tired skin. You need to pick the right color for your skin (nothing too orange or shimmery). Brush it on anywhere the sun would normally hit—your cheeks, forehead, nose, and chin. To fake it with self-tanner, start with clean skin that has nothing on it. I like to do it at night before I go to bed because then I wake up in the morning looking better. Apply it all over your face, but keep it away from your eyes. The real trick is to apply a little to your neck and on your ears—that way it will all blend in. Don't apply too much at once. I'd much rather put an extra coat on in an hour if it didn't do very much than have it come out too dark and unnatural-looking. And don't forget to wash your hands! Stained palms (or the area in between fingers) are a telltale sign of a novice self-tanner. If you use self-tanner on your body, be really careful to get it all around—you might not see the back of your body, but everyone else does. For mistakes—too dark a shade or an obvious streak—you can help it fade faster by exfoliating with a body scrub in the shower. Remember that you might need two colors—one for the summer and a lighter shade for the winter.

Moisturize, moisturize, moisturize. Hydration is key when you're not feeling or looking good. Drink lots of water and put lots of moisture on your skin. A rich moisturizer can take years away from your face the way it smooths everything out. Don't be afraid of goo! Unless, of course, you have really oily skin, but then consider yourself lucky because your skin already has that youthful sheen women with dry skin are always trying to re-create.

Scent yourself. Something as simple as a spritz of fragrance can lift your mood and make you feel better on a bad day. Or try a little aromatherapy. You can use scented candles, essential oils applied straight to your skin or in your bath, or even a sprinkle of powder that's laced with essential oil. Different scents will have different effects: Lavender can be very soothing when you're feeling stressed, and peppermint in the morning will wake you up and make you feel more energized. I love rose essential oil because it makes me think of my grandmother who always wore rose. Scent can be a very powerful memory trigger, so it's good to find one that makes you think of a fond memory.

Don't forget concealer. This is the day you need the right concealer more than ever. If you've got really dark circles, it might not be able to cover them completely, but it will help! Just be sure to get it into the inner corners of the eyes (to open them up a bit), and skip the powder on top if your skin is feeling extra dry. (See chapter 16 for more application tricks.)

Blush your cheeks. I firmly believe that when you're having a bad beauty day, putting on too much makeup is a huge mistake. You think it will help disguise how you feel, but the truth is, it often makes you look worse. What does help? A light touch of blush. Pick a nice, warm pink tone that instantly wakes up your face.

Curl your lashes. The most tired eyes look more open and awake when you curl your lashes (even if you don't put mascara on afterward). The secret is to clamp the curler over your lashes and then close your eye and hold it for ten seconds.

Hide behind glasses. A good, stylish pair of frames comes in handy when you're having a bad day. When I'm extra sleepy, I slip on glasses to help hide my telltale tired eyes. And if you are wearing glasses, skip most of the eye makeup. A bit of mascara is enough to help liven up eyes.

Get some exercise. Getting your blood pumping is a sure way to make yourself look, and feel, better. Even if you can only sneak in a quick walk around the block, it will help bring color to your face. I find that after a good workout I hardly need any makeup for hours.

Take a bath. Giving yourself twenty minutes in the tub—preferably filled with some wonderfully fragrant aromatherapy oils—is one of the best ways to get revitalized.

Get a blowout. If the problem is a bad hair day, it's worth the time and money to get your hair washed and blown out by a professional. You can often walk into a salon without an appointment—and walk out half an hour later looking and feeling much, much better.

Try sheer, glossy, nude lips. When you want to look more pulled together—but don't really have the time to do it—put on a lipstick or gloss that has just enough color to highlight your lips and add a soft shine. And remember, nude doesn't mean pale; it means a color that's close to your lips' natural shade.

Eat some chocolate. Okay, maybe eating a piece of chocolate won't help you look better on a bad beauty day, but it will make you feel better! Indulge yourself a little.

And when all else fails, don't fight it. Just realize you're having a bad day and go with it. Chances are, you'll feel (and look) better tomorrow!

IF YOU'RE SICK, trying to wear too much makeup will only make you look worse. What you do want: a lot of moisture and a little bit of color. When you've got a cold or the flu, the skin around your nose naturally gets dry and red (no matter how soft the tissues are, all that blowing still takes a toll on your skin). You might want to use something heavier than your usual moisturizer to combat this—a super-emollient eye balm or even a dab of Vaseline—and then cover the red with a bit of stick foundation (and bring it with you for touch-ups throughout the day). Add a little bit of pink blush to cheeks and sheer lip gloss or balm, but skip the eye makeup (just a coat of mascara is enough).

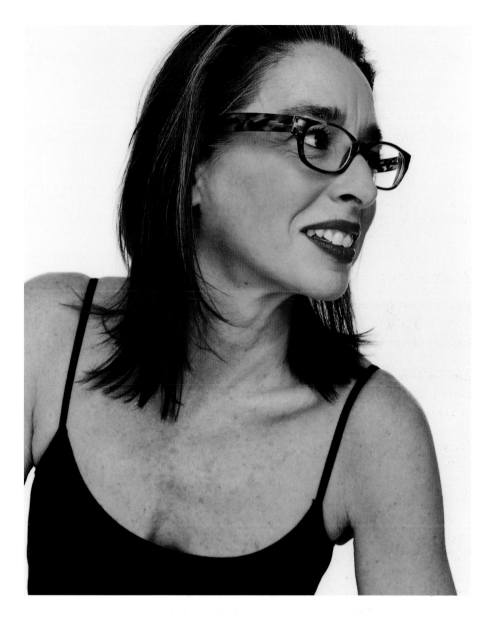

A good, stylish pair of frames come in handy when you're having a bad day.

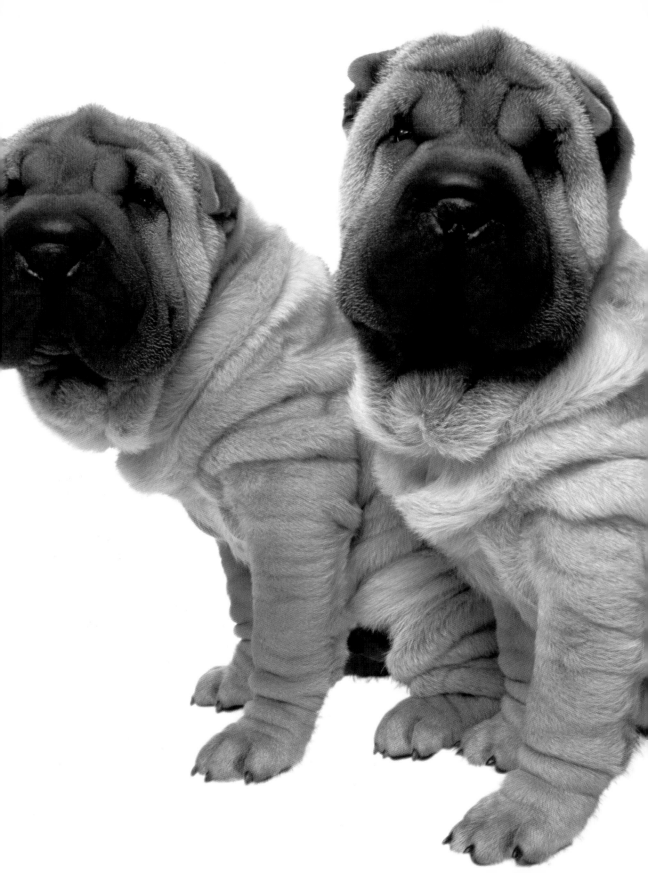

25 LINES, LINES, LINES:
LEARNING TO LOVE THEM
(OR HOW TO LOSE THEM)

I like lines in a woman's face. My role models are the women who wear their lines on their faces with pride. I remember a moment when I was just over thirty, and I saw a gorgeous black-and-white photo of Debra Winger. She was smiling a huge smile, and I noticed these awesome little lines around her eyes. And for the first time I thought, Okay, I can do this age thing, and it can look really good. The fact is, lines belong on our faces. They're nothing more than the result of moving our faces, showing emotions, reacting and expressing ourselves. That's why they're called smile lines, laugh lines, expression lines, even frown lines—because they come naturally from doing all of those things. Of course, even though you can't really fight the effects of the years, you can help by protecting skin from the environment. (See chapter 13 for sunscreen tips.)

Bobbi's Line-Friendly Makeup Tricks
Yes, I believe that lines on the face can be beautiful, but as with every feature on our faces, we can use makeup in subtle ways to make them more flattering:

- Make sure skin is well hydrated. Regular exfoliation (with a gentle scrub or an AHA cream) will help skin shed dry layers. But there's nothing better than adding serious moisture to the skin—it literally plumps up the skin to fill lines out a bit.
- Stick to cream formulas for your concealer, foundation, and blush. They'll help further hydrate skin; plus they're less likely to fall into lines and call more attention to them.
- Add a bit of color on your cheeks. Try a cream blush topped with just a touch of powder blush to help it last; it will soften your overall appearance.
- For lines around the lips, the key is to keep them moist. Use a rich lip balm or even eye cream to smooth on lips and around the mouth. Don't try to cover the lines with foundation. Instead choose a creamy lipstick and a matching lip liner to keep color from creeping off lips and into lines.

What Can a Doctor Do?

There are a number of nonsurgical techniques that let you reverse signs of age without having to commit to more invasive plastic surgery, many of which can be done in no longer than a lunch hour. But as with most things, moderation is the key. A little fix can go a long way—making sure your face still looks like you, only a bit better. Also, bear in mind that none of these fixes come cheap; while prices vary depending on where you live, you can expect to pay up to several hundred dollars for any of these treatment options. Dermatologist Dr. Jeanine Downie explains: "It really is possible to look younger with many of these noninvasive techniques. I'm not saying that you'll be able to erase all the years off your face, but you will be able to erase a few!" Here are some options she gives to her patients.

Chemical peels. A doctor applies a chemical solution to the face that causes an effect similar to a sunburn. Over the course of a few days, the skin will blister and peel off, revealing new, less-wrinkled, skin underneath. Younger women, with less sun damage to their skin, can get a series of six to ten (once a month) milder peels that will simply exfoliate dead skin to make lines look less noticeable and skin tone more even. They will then need to get a peel three to four times a year to maintain the results.

Pros: There's nothing better for smoothing skin texture and improving tone. Peels will also help fade fine lines.

Cons: They can irritate the skin if left on too long, and if the peel is administered by an inexperienced person, it can lead to permanent scarring and pigment alterations.

Laser resurfacing. Lasers are light pumps that emit high-intensity light radiation that can literally vaporize the targeted skin as well as stimulate the skin's own collagen production to increase firmness and elasticity. Laser resurfacing can be used to reduce or remove lines, erase age spots, treat scars, and remove tattoos. It's better for people with light complexions because it can cause uneven pigment in darker skin. This procedure usually lasts from three to five years. Many doctors offer light "lunchtime lasers," but it really takes more than those can do to make a noticeable difference on deep lines or very dark patches.

Pros: Laser treatments can erase significant sun damage.

Cons: You have to expect some purplish bruising on the treated area for seven to ten days. For women who choose to do full-face resurfacing, you may be pink for three to six months after the procedure.

Botox. Short for botulinum toxin, this is the same agent that causes botulism food poisoning. But used in tiny purified amounts and injected into a targeted facial muscle, Botox is capable of immobilizing the muscle. The result: If it's injected into the area between your eyebrows, for example, the muscle that makes you frown will be paralyzed. And if you can't make that furrow, the wrinkle there will soften and fade. It is, however, a temporary solution; the immobilizing effects of the Botox last only about three to four months. It's most commonly used on the forehead and on crow's-feet around the eyes.

Pros: There's very little bruising; it's an easy and quick fix.

Cons: Since the treatment lasts only a few months, this can become an expensive addiction. Also, since the needle has to be inserted directly into the muscle, it is painful (if only for a few seconds). It is rare, but it is possible for your lid to droop temporarily (lasting approximately two weeks). Therefore, it is important to keep your head upright for four hours after treatment.

Collagen. This is the protein substance that gives skin its firmness. Our bodies naturally produce it, but as we get older, our skin has less and less (which is why skin looks less full and plump than it did when you were younger). Most of the collagen used to fill in lines is derived from cows. Normally, a series of collagen injections is necessary to fill out lines, and the results last about four months. (A new more permanent synthetic type of collagen called Artecoll is currently being tested.)

Pros: The results are instant.

Cons: You need to have it done by someone who is an expert in collagen injecting; serious complications (like hitting a blood vessel) can occur with less-experienced practitioners.

Dermabrasion: The doctor uses a rapidly rotating metal brush to remove the skin surface, making it an effective way to treat acne or chickenpox scars as well as fine lines and uneven skin pigment. After treatment, skin will be very red and swollen, but it should heal completely in about two to three weeks. Since the new skin that's exposed after dermabrasion is very sensitive, you have to avoid the sun for several months posttreatment. For less serious skin surface problems, there is a milder version of the same process, called microdermabrasion. It can remove fine lines, but they will eventually recur.

Pros: It evens out small areas of bad scarring.

Cons: There is a risk of infection and the possibility that the treated area won't match the pigment on the rest of the face.

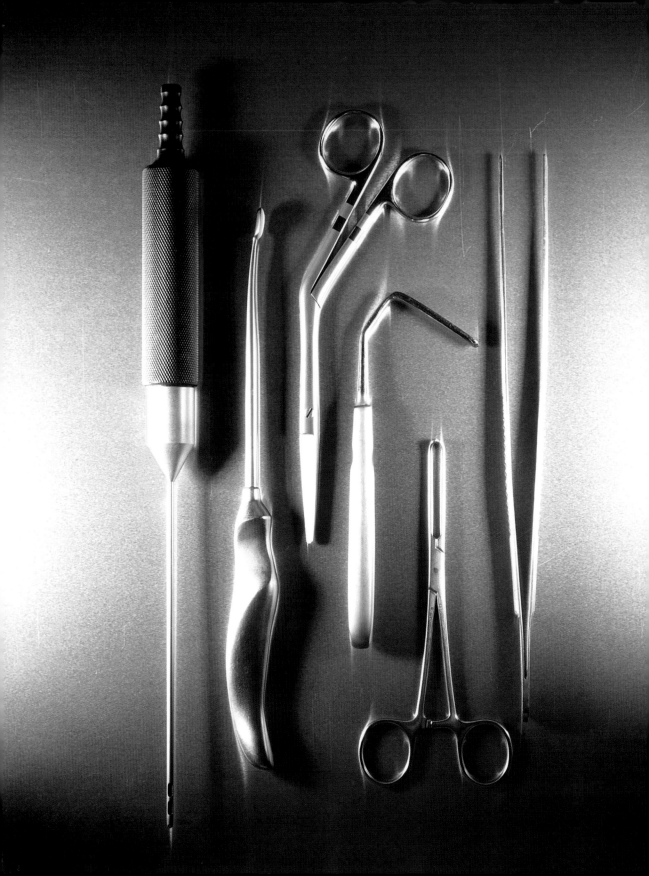

26 PLASTIC SURGERY:
WHAT YOU NEED TO KNOW

I won't come out and say that I'm completely against plastic surgery. But I'm not completely in favor of it either. I think it's great that it's out there as an option, and I've seen it do wonders for some people. However, I've also seen too many women who look like they've had plastic surgery. There's a fine line between making a big improvement and having a fake, unnatural, and tight look. The bottom line is that if you decide to have any kind of plastic surgery, you cannot expect the end result to be perfect. You will have scars, you might have a painful recovery, and you might not love what the new you looks like. These are all things to consider carefully before you choose to get plastic surgery.

If we could get more used to ourselves naturally aging, we'd feel a lot better about ourselves and not be running off to the plastic surgeon at the first hint of a wrinkle. I understand that erasing signs of age can be important for actresses, newscasters, and other people whose faces are their livelihoods (which is why I'm thankful that's not the case in my career!). But be careful not to look at these women on TV and think they are ideals of aging beautifully. They do look amazing, but when you see them in person (especially without makeup), they often look like they've had a lot of plastic surgery. So just remember that whenever you do something as radical as plastic surgery, most people are going to know you've done some-thing—they aren't going to believe that it's simply a new haircut that's transformed you!

> There's a fine line between making a big improvement and just looking fake, unnatural, and tight.

I'm not going to tell you not to have plastic surgery. I'm just saying that you need to think about your options and go there only as a last resort. Do your research, know the pros and the cons, don't rush into anything, and have realistic expectations about what the results will look like. Also, know that sometimes the right makeup can fix what you perceive as flaws and might make you change your mind about having surgery.

Makeup Tips That Are as Good as Surgery

- **Moisturize!** Keeping skin well hydrated will make it look fuller, plumper, and less saggy (plus smooth out some fine lines).
- **Go creamy.** Toss anything in your makeup bag that's oil-free, and cut down on powder-formula blushes and eye shadows. Cream makeup will blend more easily into skin, calling less attention to lines.
- **Wear blush.** A little color can add lift to the cheeks.
- **Contour your eyes.** The right eye makeup application can help counteract droopy eyelids. Avoid using dark shadow all over the lid and stick to more neutral shades; then highlight with bone shadow under the brows to lift eyes and make them appear more wide open.
- **When in doubt, distract.** If forehead lines bother you, play up your eyes. If crow's-feet drive you crazy, then skip the heavy eye makeup and wear a nice glossy lip color to bring focus away from your eyes.

Do Your Homework: What You Need to Know Before Signing On with a Surgeon

- Don't rely on a friend's recommendation. Although it's always helpful to talk to a friend about her experience with a certain doctor, her results are no guarantee that yours will be similar. Also, don't be swayed by the fact the doctor has been quoted in lots of glossy magazines. That may mean the doctor does good work, or it may mean the doctor hired a good PR person. The key is to do your own research.
- Don't be sold on price alone. Plastic surgery can be very expensive, and it probably won't pay to go with the surgeon who tries to undercut the competition. On the other hand, high-end prices are not necessarily a guarantee of great results.
- Find out if the doctor you're considering is certified by the American Board of Plastic Surgery (ABPS). You can find out by calling the American Society for Aesthetic Plastic Surgery (an organization of ABPS-certified surgeons who specialize in cosmetic procedures) at (888) 272-7711.
- Ask if the doctor has hospital privileges at a nearby facility. Even if you will be having your procedure done in the doctor's office, it's

important to find out if she has operating privileges at a hospital for the same procedure you are having. That would mean that the hospital review committee has evaluated the surgeon's training and competency.

- Ask the doctor how often she performs the procedure you want to have as well as what training she has had in new techniques.
- Find out about all of the possible risks and how often they occur, as well as what your recovery will be like.
- Discuss how the doctor deals with postsurgery revisions. Find out what costs you would be responsible for if you need additional surgery.

Diary of a Face-lift: One Woman's Journey Through Plastic Surgery
When Judy Kaufman was in her mid-fifties, she started thinking about having a face-lift. She was unhappy with the way she looked, especially the sagging skin under her chin and the lines around her eyes and mouth. This is her story.

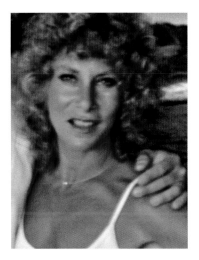

Judy in her thirties (above), a time where she thought she looked her best, and Judy before surgery (right).

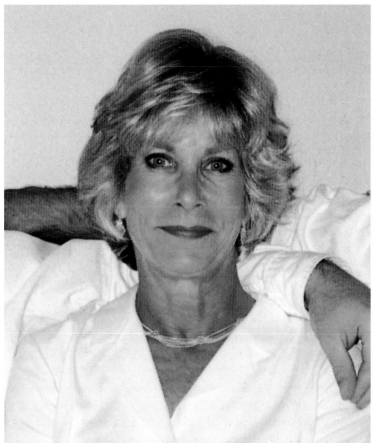

Before Surgery

I got several names of doctors and talked to other women who'd had the procedure done. I saw three or four doctors for consultations. But I felt like I had to find a doctor who I really clicked with. I wanted to feel comfortable and not just go with the one with the best resume. In retrospect, that may have been a mistake.

I booked the appointment for the surgery six months in advance. During the pre-op visits I told the doctor exactly what I wanted. I told him I didn't want to look like I'd had a face-lift, and that I was concerned about the deep wrinkles around my eyes. He tried to talk me into a brow lift, but I rejected that. We agreed that he'd use a laser to treat the wrinkles around my mouth and eyes.

The Operation

I had the surgery done in the hospital, and I had to spend one night there. The doctor made incisions behind and above both of my ears and under my chin. He pulled the skin back and sliced off the excess. When he was finished, I had stitches under my chin and behind my ears and staples in the incisions above my ears. Granted I was knocked out on anesthesia and pain medication, so I can't say I was actually ever in any pain. I healed very quickly and very well. The stitches and staples came out after a week. There were almost no bruises, the swelling went down quickly, and I was looking and feeling pretty normal after about two weeks.

The Results

Overall, I wasn't happy with the way it turned out. I still have lines around my mouth. I didn't like the way he did the bottom of my chin—I thought it looked uneven. So I went back to the doctor and told him all of the things I was unhappy about. He said he would need to open up all the incisions again. He would do it in the office, but I would still have to pay for the anesthesia and medical supplies. Then it occurred to me that if I'm not happy with what he did, why should I trust him to go back and do more? So I plan to go to a good dermatological surgeon instead to have deep laser around my mouth, which will hopefully get rid of the lines.

The fact is, I don't think anyone would ever look at me and think I had anything done. And I don't mean that in a good way! I mean that I literally don't look any different. Looking back, some of it was my own mistake. Even though I did a lot of research, I think that I chose the wrong doctor by going with the one I felt I had the best rapport with instead of the one most well known for the procedure. It just goes to show that there really are no guarantees, and that it's impossible to know how you will look after your surgery.

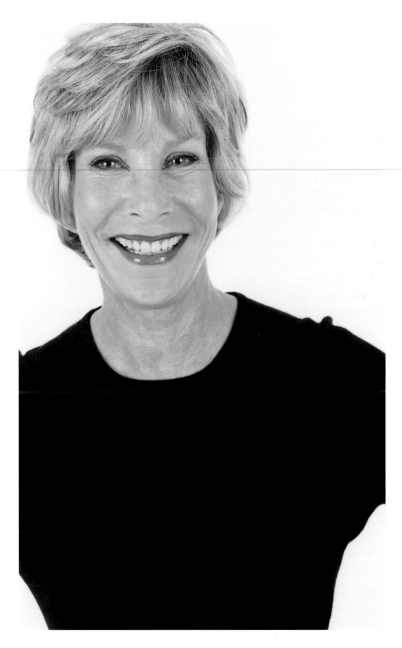

Judy Kaufman after her facelift.

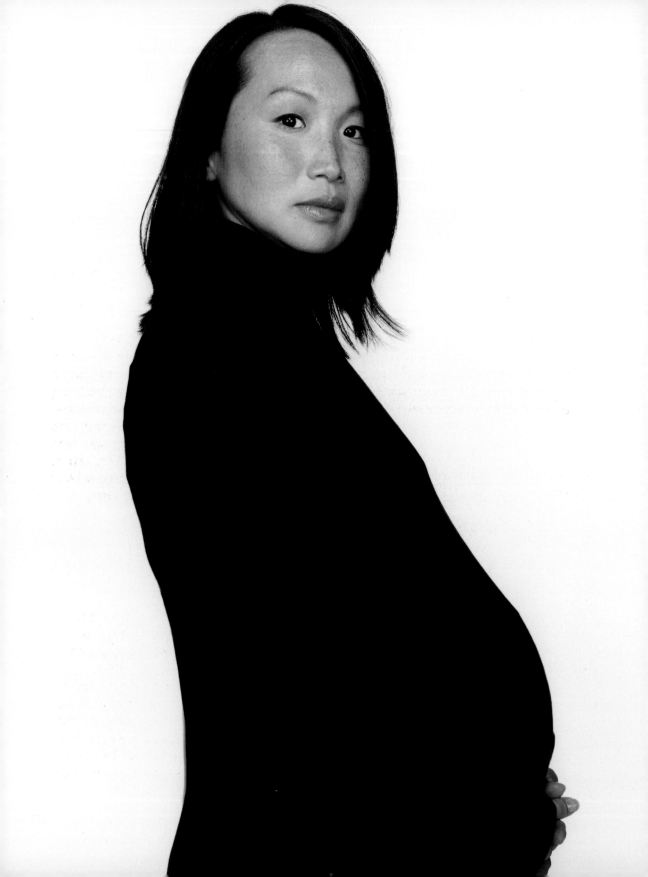

27 THE BEAUTY OF HAVING A BABY

When you're pregnant, makeup becomes crucial because it's one of the few things you can actually take charge of. You're not in complete control of how your body looks, how your brain works, or how you feel, but you can be in control of your makeup. This is why now is a nice time to treat yourself to some new cosmetics. You might not be spending a lot of money on clothes, so pamper yourself a little with makeup, manicures, pedicures—anything that's going to make you feel better.

While you're pregnant, your hormones take over big time! This will affect not only your mood but also your looks. Skin can become oilier or drier than normal, so you need to adjust your routine accordingly. When I was pregnant, my skin became extremely dry. So I added lots of oil—to the bath, all over my body after a shower, and on my face and hair. (Yes, hair changes during pregnancy and after the baby's born, too.) Some women experience pimples, even if they haven't broken out in years. All of this is perfectly normal (although certainly frustrating!). Just try not to fret about any of it too much because all these hormonal changes will go away.

Pay a little extra attention to your skin and really pamper yourself.

During your pregnancy is a good time to pay a little extra attention to your skin and really pamper yourself. Treat yourself to a luxurious body cream and really use it. After every shower, apply it to damp skin, and let it absorb. Don't forget about your feet; a little cream can do wonders for worn-out feet. I love using scented cream, but you may find that your sensitivity to smell (also hormone related) will make this a turnoff. Even your favorite perfume might not smell good for the moment, so switch to something lighter or try using an essential oil (lavender and grapefruit smell great together). I loved using special baby creams and lotions while I was pregnant. To me that smell just reminds me of a baby, and I think it's part of the ritual of mentally preparing. Even now, I often use a baby lotion and it brings me back to the memory of that special time (plus, they are wonderful for keeping skin soft).

Here are tips on how to cope with a few of the other curveballs your body throws you during those nine months.

Stretch marks. You can rub all the cocoa butter, oil, or special "stretch mark creams" you want onto your belly and breasts, but you might get stretch marks anyway, especially if your mom or sister has them. Keeping your skin moisturized certainly can't hurt, but it won't necessarily prevent marks altogether. If it's your first baby, you'll probably freak out about them more, but after the baby's born, they will become less important. Your priorities change, and it's the baby you worry about more than your stretch marks!

Line of demarcation. This appears on your belly, from pubic bone to belly button, usually sometime during your second trimester. It's caused by hormonal influences on your skin pigment (darker-skinned women may see a more pronounced line), and fortunately, it will normally fade away after the baby is born.

It's the baby you worry about more than stretch marks!

Dry, brittle nails. This is a very common problem because the baby grabs your nutrients first. Be sure you're eating plenty of protein and calcium to compensate. Apply a rich cuticle oil every night, and keep hand cream in your purse, in your desk drawer, or next to the kitchen sink, and use it often throughout the day.

Sun protection. Your skin is extra sensitive during pregnancy, so be vigilant about sunscreen. This is especially important to help cope with the pigment changes your skin is experiencing (thanks to your hormones), such as the so-called mask of pregnancy. This darkened skin often appears around the cheeks, nose, and eyes, and sun exposure will only make it more obvious.

Now, More Than Ever, Take These Simple Beauty Rules to Heart

1. Be gentle and kind to yourself.
2. Pay attention to what your skin and body need.
3. No one's perfect—just do your best.
4. This too shall pass.

And to quote my friend Ann Curry, "Don't be hard on yourself while you're pregnant—remember the big, important job your body is doing."

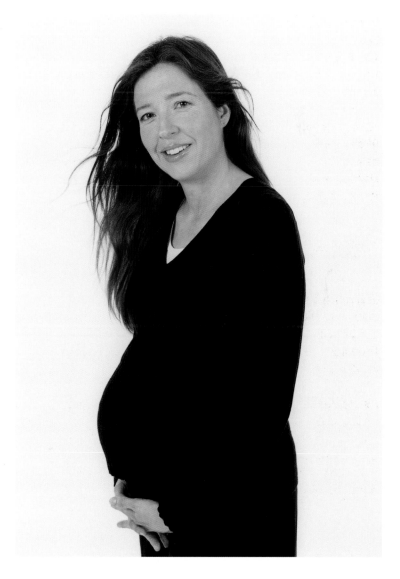

After the Baby's Born

Now is when it really gets tough to find any time to take care of yourself. I'm always amazed when I see a mom who's got perfectly blow-dried hair. When my kids were first born, I'd find myself still not even having showered at four in the afternoon, let alone done my hair or put on any makeup. You're going to need things to be as simple and fast as possible, so think of things that save time. Keep a bottle of body oil in the shower to throw on so you can skip moisturizer; get some gel that you can put in your hair and not need to blow it dry (and thank God for ponytails!). And for your makeup, get a palette and create your own all-in-one makeup kit. Put a concealer, some cream blush, two lipsticks, and a lip balm in it. That way you can do your makeup in a minute without even having to find different products. It's not about putting on a lot of makeup, but just enough to make you feel fresher and more pulled together. If that means just concealer and lip gloss, then just do that. You'll look better and, more importantly, feel better about yourself.

Quick Fixes and Dual-Purpose Products

- All-in-one face palette
- SPF 15 tinted moisturizer
- SPF lipsticks
- Chubby pencils to use on lips or cheeks
- Moisturizing balm for face, hands, cuticles, and more
- Scented lotions and oils

Babying Your Newborn's Skin

A baby's skin is so much more delicate than ours, so don't even think about using any adult products to wash or moisturize your newborn. Find the gentlest cleanser (one formulated just for babies is your best bet) and use it to clean the baby's hair and body. Make sure you pick one that's not really sudsy—you want to be able to rinse the baby clean without too much effort. Also, think about things that will make bathing the baby easier, such as cleansers in safe plastic bottles and pump dispensers you can use with one hand. Be sure that whatever you use to wash your baby smells good or is unscented; you want that good baby smell, not a strong perfumey scent. After a bath, moisturize your baby's skin by massaging in some baby oil. Not only will it keep the skin soft, but massaging your baby is a wonderful bonding experience for both of you.

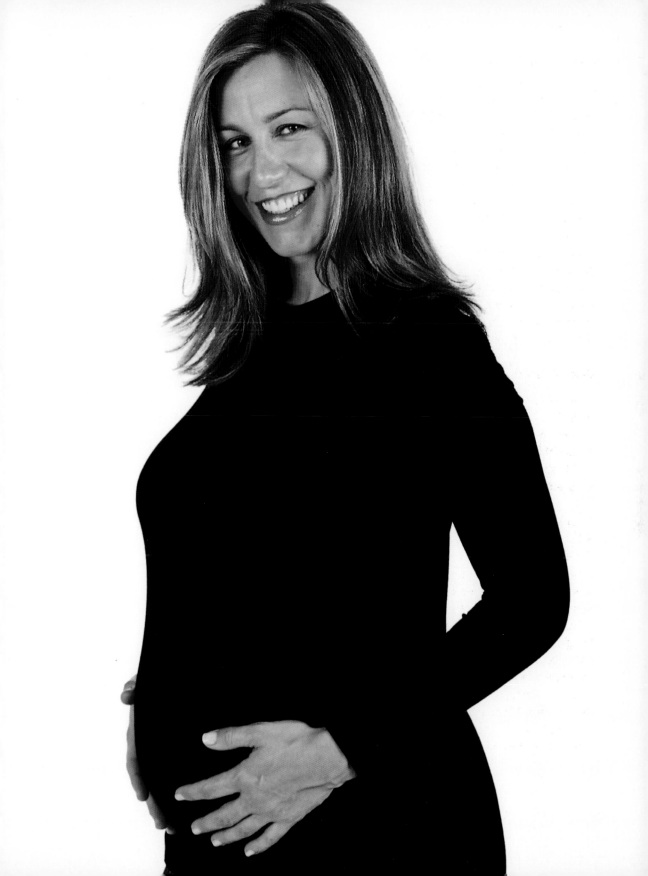

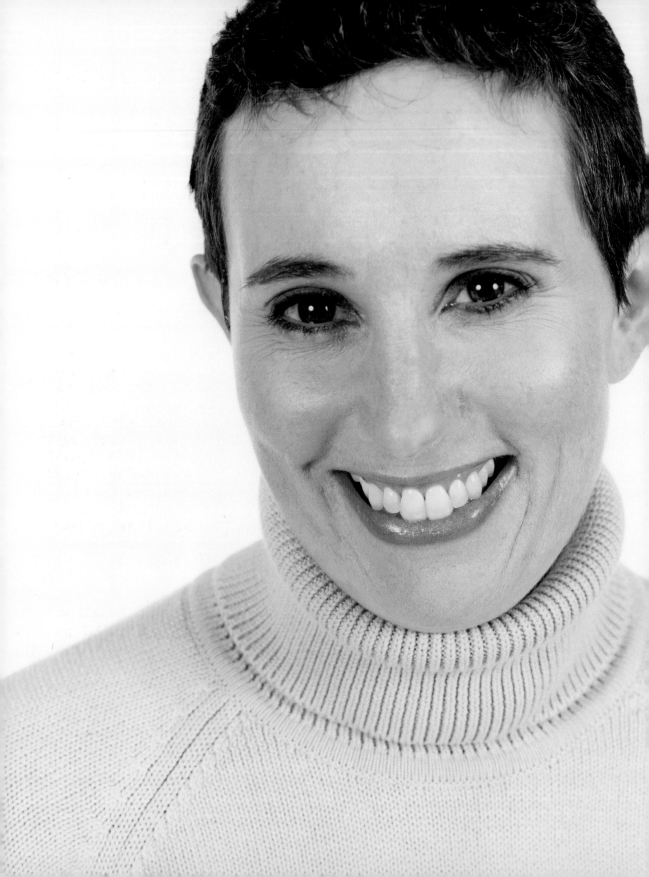

28 COPING WITH CANCER...BEAUTIFULLY

When you are battling a serious illness, you are obviously concerned first and foremost with regaining your health. But even at a time when getting better is your top priority, looking better can have an enormous impact on your self-confidence, your outlook, and your emotional well-being. For women who are coping with chemotherapy treatments, the effect the treatments can have on their looks—and how that makes them feel about themselves—can be nearly as devastating as the disease itself.

Now is not the time to abandon your beauty routine entirely, nor is it the time to go overboard with makeup. Your body, your hair, and your skin are going through some significant changes that your beauty routine will need to address. But it's important to remember that these changes are temporary and that your illness doesn't define who you are as a woman. When you finish going through chemotherapy, your hair will grow back, your eyebrows and eyelashes will reappear, and your skin tone and texture will return to the way they used to be. In the meantime, there are several beauty tricks and makeup techniques you can use to look your best and feel like yourself again. One of my makeup artists, Suzette Rodriguez-Waller, works with many women going through this tough transition. Here, she shares what she has learned.

Skin Care Concerns

The most important step you can take in caring for your face is recognizing that your skin has changed and treating it accordingly. Chances are, chemotherapy has left your skin looking and feeling extremely dry—maybe even red, flaky, or scaly—and sensitive. The solution is to find the richest, gentlest cream you can; natural hydrating ingredients like shea butter and glycerine will soothe and soften without irritating your skin. And for the areas that tend to get especially dry, such as around the eyes and nose, I would recommend an extra-rich eye cream or balm.

Pamela Scott, breast cancer survivor.

183

Makeup: A Little Goes a Long Way

Think of your makeup as a veil of color for your face, not a mask. Trying to pile on layers of foundation, too much blush, and heavy eye shadow isn't the answer. Once your face is well moisturized, start by using a bit of concealer to help hide dark under-eye circles. If your old concealer doesn't seem to be doing the job, it's probably because the color is no longer right for your skin tone. (See chapter 16 for tips on selecting the right shade and application techniques.) Your concealer will need to have a yellow undertone, especially now that your skin may be slightly more sallow than it is naturally. Once you have the right shade and enough moisture around your eyes, the concealer will blend effortlessly into your skin. After that, it's time for foundation. If your skin tone is looking uneven, you may need to wear a full face of foundation, but that doesn't mean you have to cake it on. The goal of foundation isn't to add color to the skin (that's where blush comes in), but to smooth it out and make it look even. Then you can use blush or bronzer, with a light touch, to give your skin back its healthy glow. (See chapter 18 for blush tips.) Your lips may also be feeling extremely dry, so now is not the time to experiment with matte lipsticks. Apply a liberal coat of moisturizing lip balm and then a little bit of creamy lipstick or gloss in whatever shade makes you feel pretty.

Eyebrows and Lashes: Creating an Illusion

Losing your hair—which includes your eyebrows and lashes—can be one of the most traumatic side effects of chemotherapy. Even women who have hardly worn any makeup their entire lives suddenly feel naked and like they need a little something to make them feel prettier. Regardless of whether or not you choose to wear a wig, using the right makeup to re-create your eyebrows and lashes can make a huge difference in the appearance of your face.

Creating eyebrows. Choose a shade of powdered eye shadow that matches your wig (if you choose to wear one) or compliments your eyes. Just be careful not to go too dark—slate, sable, and mahogany are better choices than charcoal or black. Take the powder on an eyebrow brush and stamp it bit by bit (don't brush it on) into your skin where your natural brow would be. Even if there is no hair there at the moment, you can see where the brow was and just follow that arch.

Creating the illusion of eyelashes. Using false eyelashes is a wonderful option for special occasions, although the application may be too time-consuming for everyday. An easy technique for faking the

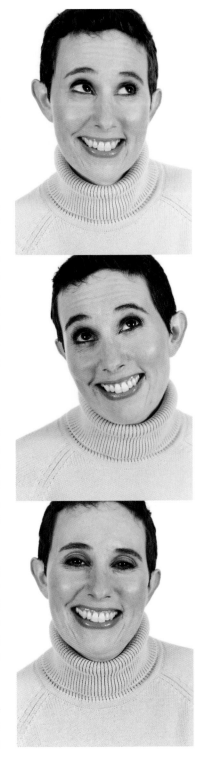

appearance of lashes is to take an eyeliner brush (you can use it wet or dry); dip it into a dark brown, gray, or charcoal shadow; and stamp it into the lash line. Using a dark color shadow helps create the illusion of hair being there, so it looks like more than just eyeliner.

Where to Go for Help

- **The Looking Glass:** This beauty workshop, started by Bobbi Brown and makeup artist Suzette Rodriguez-Waller, is a free program held at Gilda's Club (a cancer support center named for comedian Gilda Radner who died of ovarian cancer) in New York City and Hackensack, N.J. For information, call (212) 647-9700.
- **Look Good . . . Feel Better:** This is a free nationwide program designed to help women with cancer deal with appearance-related concerns and questions. It is sponsored by the American Cancer Society; the Cosmetic, Toiletry, and Fragrance Association; and the National Cosmetology Association. For information or to locate a program near you, call (800) 395-LOOK or log on to their web site at www.lookgoodfeelbetter.org.
- ***Beauty & Cancer:*** In this book (published by Taylor Publishing Company), Diane Doan Noyes and Peggy Mellody, R.N., deal with the special needs of women coping with the effects that cancer has on their appearance.
- **Cancer and Careers:** For helpful information on balancing your treatment and your work life (including makeup tips and beauty advice for working women with cancer), log on to www.cancerandcareers.org.

"I never felt that I didn't look beautiful."

"Before I started chemo, I went and got all my hair cut off. I thought it would be easier that way to handle losing my hair, but it was still hard when it started falling out in handfuls in the shower. That's when I really cried. Then I got a wig. You get used to it and you go on. One positive thing about surviving cancer is that you really do appreciate what you have, how precious life is and how precious the time you have is, and you don't let little things bother you anymore. When my hair grew back, I decided to keep it short. I wanted a reminder that I'm a different person now than I was before the cancer—this hair is who I am now. I couldn't just go back to being who I was.

"Even during the worst parts of the treatment, I never felt that I didn't look beautiful. I just felt that I looked sick. And that's an important difference."—Pamela Scott, 42, breast cancer survivor

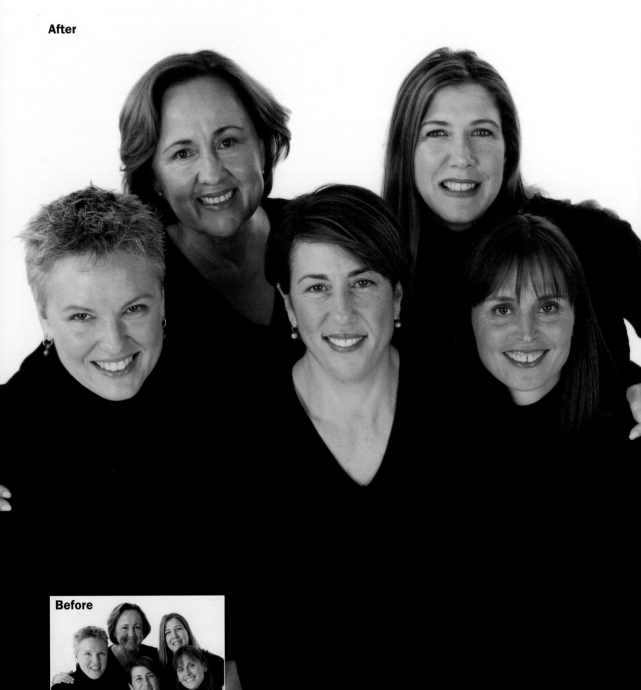

After

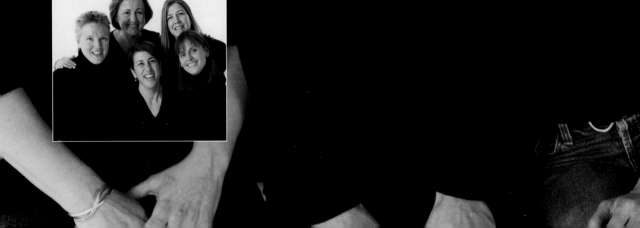

Before

29 BEAUTY BOOK GROUP:
WOMEN SHARE THEIR BEAUTY QUESTIONS, CONCERNS, AND SECRETS

What happens when you gather a group of women and ask them to talk about skin and makeup? Lots! That was the case when I turned my monthly book group meeting into a beauty question-and-answer session. I also invited my friend dermatologist Dr. Jeanine Downie, so that between the two of us we could answer all the questions the book group threw at us.

I use concealer to cover my under-eye circles, but the dark skin still shows through. And if I try to use more concealer, it looks too obviously caked on. What am I doing wrong?

You're probably using the wrong color concealer. If it's too light, it won't cover the circles and it will stand out on your skin. You want your foundation to match your skin exactly, and then the concealer should be just one shade lighter than that. Forget the ones that are green- or blue- or pink-toned—the only one that is going to cover and look natural is one with a yellow tone. Once you have the right color, you need to put it on correctly. Start with a dab of eye cream to hydrate the skin and smooth out lines (too much and the concealer will slide off, too little and the concealer will cake). Then make sure you put enough on. Most women don't use enough, so of course it doesn't really cover your circles. Put on twice as much as you want, take your finger and really pat it into your skin (no rubbing or it'll rub right off), make sure you get it into the inner corners of the eyes, and then put yellow-toned powder on top to keep it in place. On some days, when you're really tired or sick, just realize it might not help and put on very little—dark circles are better than bad concealer.

I don't have time to wear full makeup every day, but I want to be able to do just one or two things to make me look better. What should I use?

Doing one or two things is always better than nothing. What you choose is a matter of personal preference. For me, it's concealer, sheer lip color, and maybe blush. For others, it might be mascara and lip gloss. Look at your face and figure out what you want to hide or enhance. If your biggest problem is dark circles, your one thing should be concealer. If you've got small eyes, then try eye liner and mascara. If your skin looks tired and dull, brush on a little bronzer. And everyone has time to apply a quick hit of lip gloss or sheer lipstick. Pick a shade so neutral you can literally put it on as you walk out the door—no mirror required.

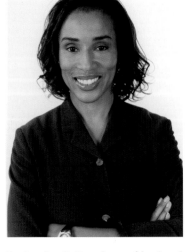

Now that I'm in my fifties, I've noticed a redness to my skin that was never there before. How can I get rid of the ruddiness?
Hormonal fluctuations can cause redness. Wearing SPF 30 every day can help decrease the redness because the condition is exacerbated by sun exposure. And you can cover it. Anything with a yellow tone will reduce the appearance of redness. So be sure that your foundation and powder both have yellow undertones. A tinted moisturizer won't give you much coverage (only foundation can do that), so it's not your best bet for disguising this problem. If you still are bothered by it, a dermatologist can prescribe a topical medication that will help reduce the redness. As a last resort, a laser can remove it by targeting the dilated blood vessels.

Dr. Jeanine B. Downie, my friend and dermatologist, shared her skin care wisdom with my book group.

For the past five years I've been wearing bangs (even though I don't think they look good on me) because I'm really self-conscious about my frown lines. What can I do to make the lines less obvious?
Without going the cosmetic surgery route, you could start wearing more eye makeup to distract from the lines that bother you. Playing up your eyes with a coat of black mascara and a neutral-colored liner will draw attention to your good features—and away from the lines. If you want to try something more drastic, the first step might be Botox injections or, if the lines are really deep, collagen. Both of these procedures can be performed in a dermatologist's or plastic surgeon's office and take less than an hour, but they are also temporary fixes and can carry unwanted side effects.

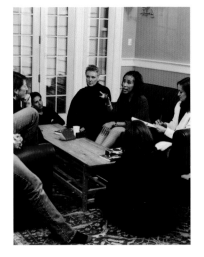

I'm forty-seven and still get clogged pores. Is it really worth the time and money to get a facial once a month?
Getting a facial can be a very pampering, relaxing experience, but you'll get more cosmetic bang for your buck at the dermatologist. If you go to the dermatologist for a glycolic acid peel (which helps skin turn over dead cells and improves skin texture, leaving the face looking smoother and less lined), the doctor can do one that has a 75 percent strength. A facialist is only licensed to use a product that has about 5 to 10 percent strength. So you might be better off

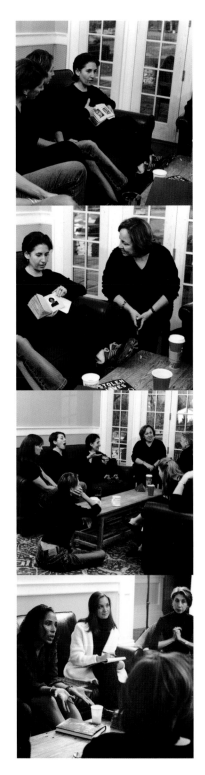

getting a massage if you crave relaxation and going to a dermatologist if you really want to see a noticeable improvement in the way your skin looks.

I'm not twenty years old anymore, but I still like to experiment with different colors of eyeliner. How do I know if I've gone too far?

Only you can really tell, and if you think it looks great, then that's half the battle. But as a rule, as you get older—unless your style is very funky and artistic—bold-colored eyeliner or mascara usually looks too trendy. If you don't want to stick with the obvious neutrals—like brown, gray, or charcoal—look for colors that have a lot of black in them. They will add some color but are still technically neutral. For example, instead of a bright blue, try a deep navy; instead of purple, try mauve; instead of green, try a more muted hunter or khaki shade.

Should I avoid shimmery or frosted makeup as I get older?

Not necessarily. Glossy lips look very youthful, and a creamy, glossy formula is a good way to keep older lips well moisturized. You do have to be careful with shimmer because it is going to make lines on your face stand out more. The key is to use just a hint of shimmer— on your nails, eyes, or lips. Don't overdo it, and don't use frosted formulas if you find that they fall into facial lines and make them look more obvious.

My eyes naturally droop a little at the sides, making me look like I'm always tired or sad. How can I do my eye makeup to help them look more lifted?

Make sure you start with concealer and powder under the eyes to brighten eyes and make them look more open. Then you will need to line the top and bottom lids, making sure you blend the shadow out to the corners of your eyes. Use a light to medium shadow on the eyelids (also blending it out to the outer corners) to help define and lift the eyes.

My lips chap easily. How can I make my lipstick last without drying out my lips even more?

Lipstick can make dry lips look drier—and even call attention to little lines around the mouth. The best solution is to use only emollient products on the lips. That could be just a balm or lip gloss. Or if you want more color, coat lips with a nongreasy balm; then line and fill them in with a lip pencil. That will give you the look of lipstick without making lips feel dry.

Putting on just a little makeup is always better than nothing.

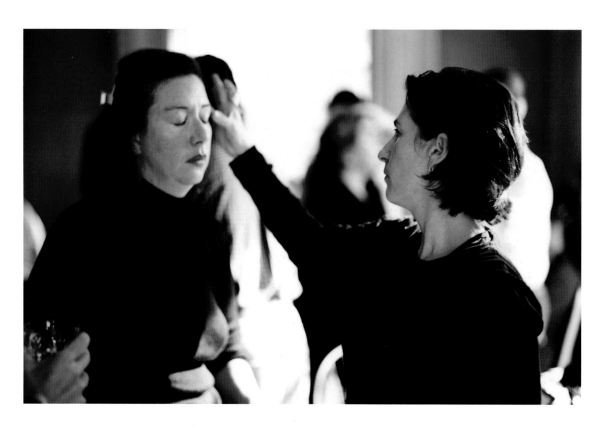

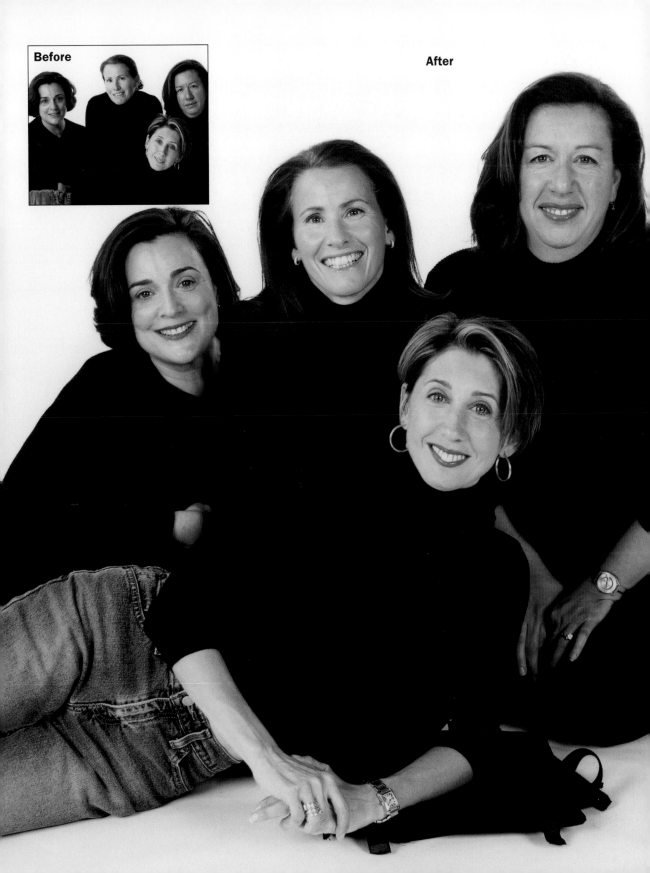

Before

After

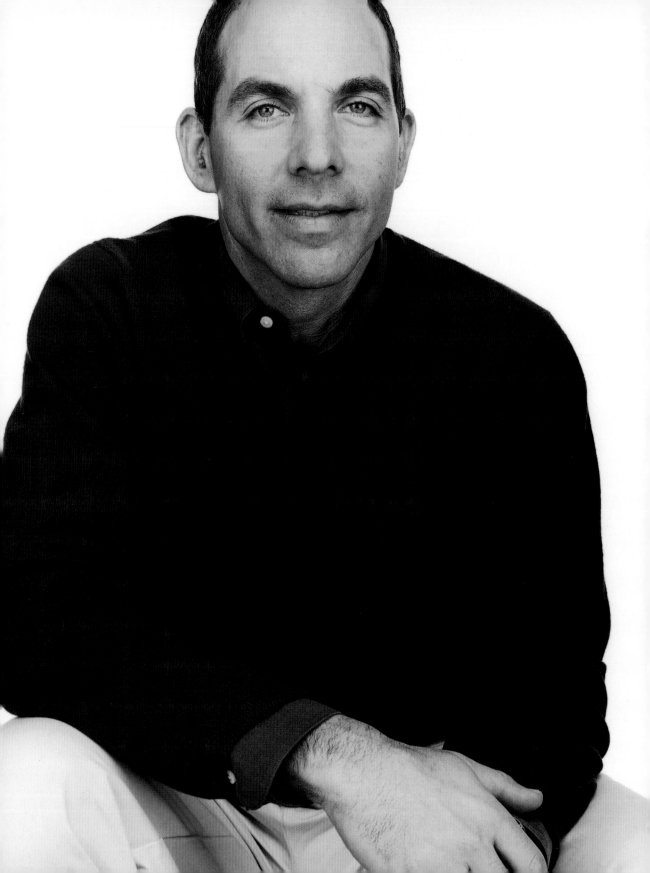

30 **A GROOMING GUIDE FOR THE MAN IN YOUR LIFE**

Most men feel that there's something unmanly about admitting that they care about their looks. But all of us who live with them—and watch them hog the bathroom mirror and steal our expensive moisturizers—know better. Men are just as concerned about their appearance as we are. The problem is that since they didn't grow up reading beauty tips in magazines, most men are fairly clueless when it comes to the topic of grooming. To help put things straight, style and grooming expert Lloyd Boston offers the answers men want to know to the grooming questions they are afraid to ask.

What's the best way to shave?
Shaving in the shower is ideal because your pores open up in the steam, and your skin and beard will be at their softest. Get a fogless shave mirror that you can hang in the shower. Use a moisturizing soap on your face and then slather on the richest, foamiest shaving cream you can find.

Most men are fairly clueless when it comes to grooming.

How can I get rid of the uni-brow look?
Symmetrical eyebrows help define the face. And the problem with the uni-brow is that it can be overpowering. You will need to practice a bit to figure out how much to take off (don't ever do too much at a time). Some guys will just have a few strays in between brows that they take out with a tweezer. (Do it after you get out of the shower and the hair will pull out less painfully.) If you have a heavy brow, you might want to have it professionally waxed or learn how to wax it yourself. But limit your hair removal just to the area between the brows. When men try to shape their eyebrows or remove hair from above or beneath them, the look is very unnatural.

My husband, Steven Plofker

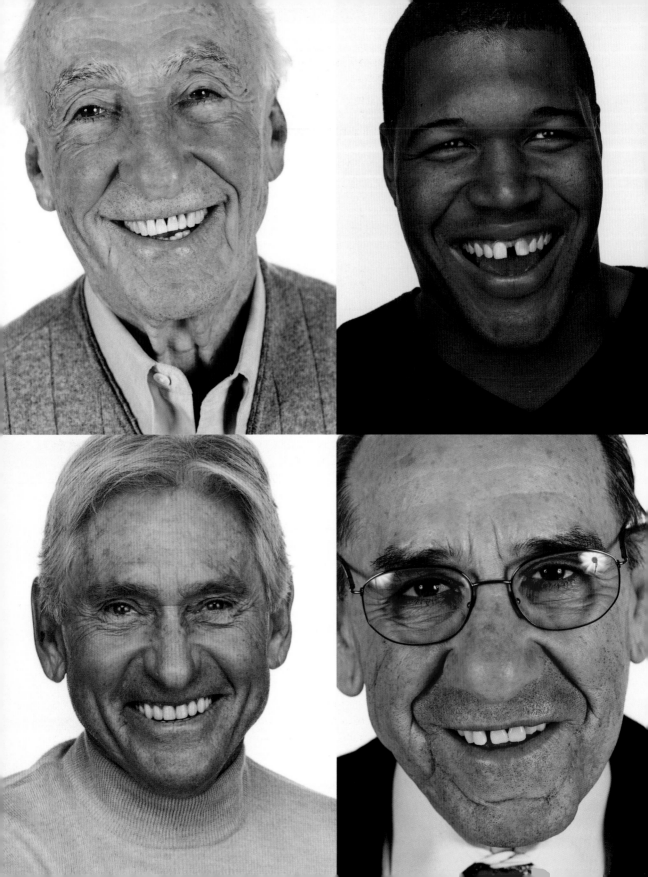

Can I trim down my unruly eyebrows?

Yes, please! Get small scissors with a blunt edge and use it to snip off eyebrow hairs that are longer than the rest. The idea isn't to cut them super-short or overly groom them, but you don't want to end up with brows that get so long they take over your entire forehead.

What's the best way to deal with nose and ear hair?

You can use the same blunt-edged scissors to trim those hairs as they pop up. And there are also special electric or battery-operated trimmers you can find at the drugstore that are designed specifically for this job.

What should I do about the hair on my chest, back, or shoulders?

First of all, you don't necessarily have to do anything about it. Some guys are just hairier than others and if you feel comfortable with it, don't worry about it. But you also need to be aware of the big picture when it comes to your appearance. You don't want to spend hundreds of dollars on a beautifully tailored suit only to have hair visibly showing at the neck of your shirt. Waxing is the way to go if you decide you do want to get rid of body hair. The trick is to find a place where you can feel comfortable having grooming treatments and establish a relationship with them. It doesn't have to be a frilly ladies' spa—you'll be surprised how many places now cater to men as well. And you should ask your barber if he can help you out. You might be surprised to find out what other services a barber can offer. Also, don't think that just because you get your chest or back waxed once, it has to become a regular event. Maybe you only wax it in the summer or just a couple of times a year to keep it from getting too out of hand.

Is there any reason to switch from the barber to a "stylist"?

That really depends on what you're looking for. If you're a simple wash-and-go guy, the $10 haircut you've been getting from the barber since you were a kid is probably fine. You might want to do a little extra homework on your own, though, to find shampoos and styling products (things your barber probably isn't up-to-date on) to make the most of your cut. But if you need more guidance about what to do with your hair—maybe you are looking for a more creative hairstyle or thinking about coloring your hair—then it would probably pay to go to a salon.

Clockwise from top left:
My friend John Cali, football star Michael Strahan, baseball legend Yogi Berra, and James Brown (my dad).

Can I get rid of the calluses on my feet without having a pedicure?

You may think there's some sort of stigma about a guy having a pedicure, but it's time to put those misconceptions aside. You'll be amazed at the difference it will make in the way your feet look and feel. (The same goes for a professional manicure.) If you think it's too feminine, think about this: There's nothing attractive, or "manly," about a ragged nail poking your significant other under the sheets! Plus, by letting a professional work on your feet—and paying close attention to the process—you can learn a few tips about how to take care of problems yourself. Namely, keep toenails trimmed short, use a pumice stone occasionally in the shower, and rub some Vaseline on your heels to soften calluses.

Can I put self-tanner on my face without looking like I'm wearing makeup?

Good grooming is all about improving your looks. But it is not about falsifying a new look. The artful use of embellishment is okay, and powerful women have known and used that for a long time. The rules for men have loosened up a bit. Most men still aren't going to wear makeup (and probably shouldn't), but there are now more and more cosmetic products that are geared specifically to men. There are self-tanning gels, tinted spot treatments for blemishes or shaving nicks, and anti-shine powders for your face to absorb excess oil. The only trick to making sure it looks natural is not over-doing it—a little embellishment can go a long, long way.

What kind of moisturizer am I supposed to use on my face?

First of all, look for one that has sunscreen in it and wear it every day to protect your skin from the harmful effects of the sun, such as skin cancer and sun-related age damage. Even if your skin isn't dry, you can look for an oil-free version that will protect your face without clogging your pores. It's also a good idea to keep a lip balm with SPF on hand—have one at home, toss one in your desk drawer, keep one in your gym bag—to make sure your lips don't get dry and cracked, especially in the winter.

Clockwise from top left:
My friend Marek Milewicz, my mentor Leonard Lauder, my son Duke, and baskeball star and friend Jason Kidd.

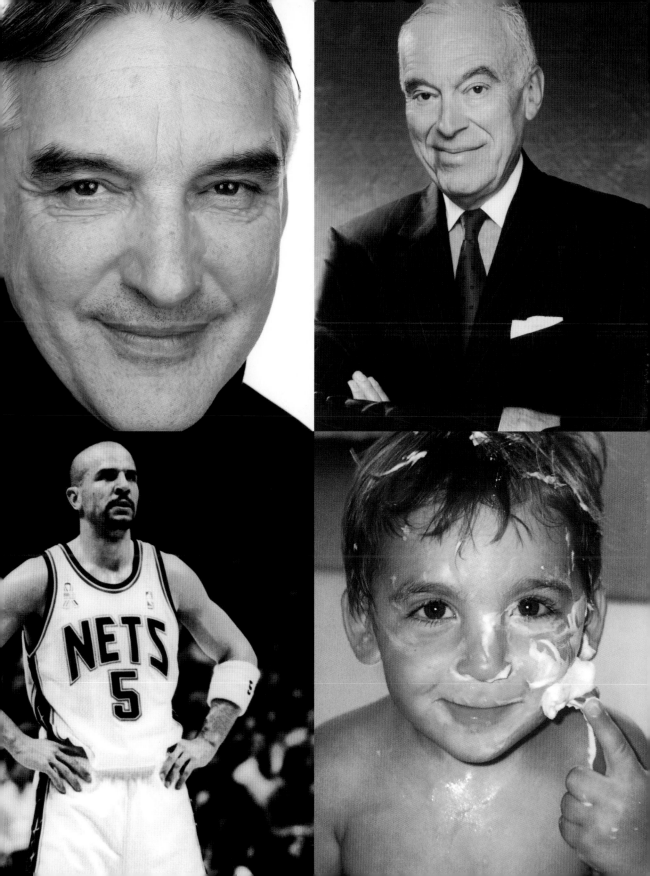

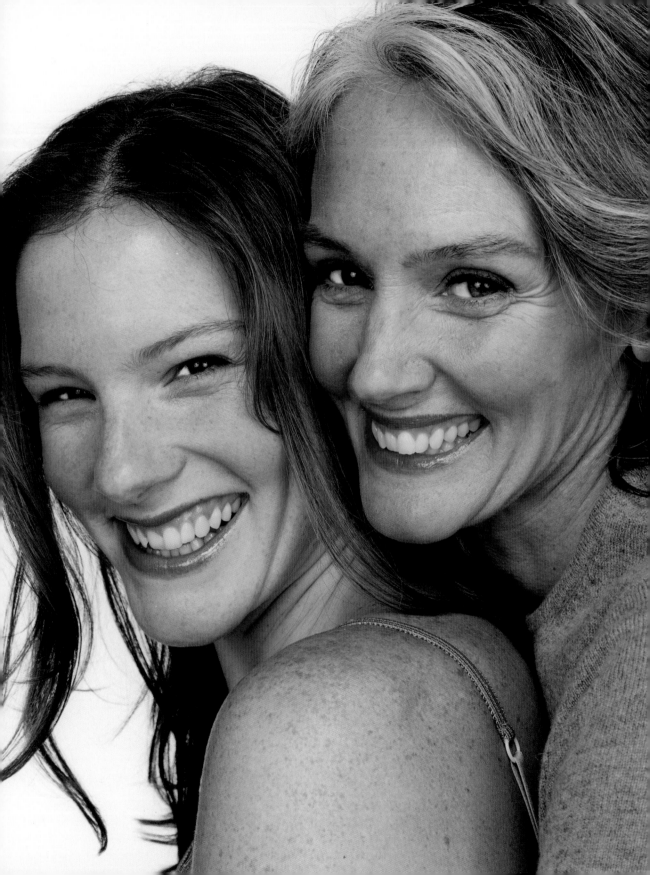

31 IT RUNS IN THE FAMILY

Mothers, daughters, aunts, sisters, grandmothers—the women in any family share a special bond. And a special beauty. Some families look so much alike it's almost eerie. If that describes yours, then you know that looking at your mom or grandmother is like looking at your own future face. Of course, there are also families who don't bear any physical resemblance to each other but share a closeness that exudes its own beauty. The best thing about families is the unconditional love and support they provide. So moms, be sure to always make your daughters feel good about themselves. Share what you know, but let them be themselves and express their beauty in their own way.

Moms, be sure to always make your daughters feel good about themselves.

Julia and her mom, Cindy.

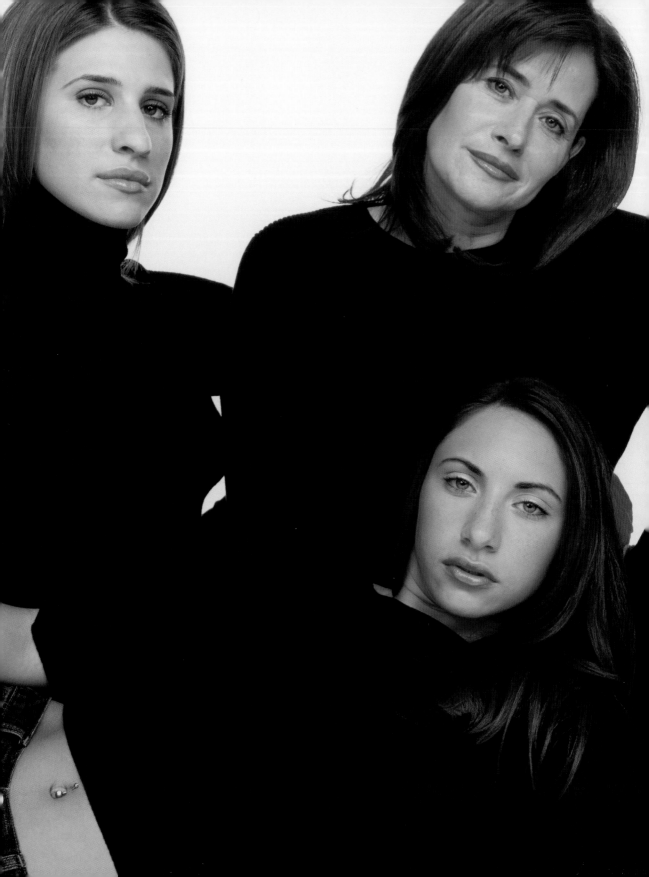

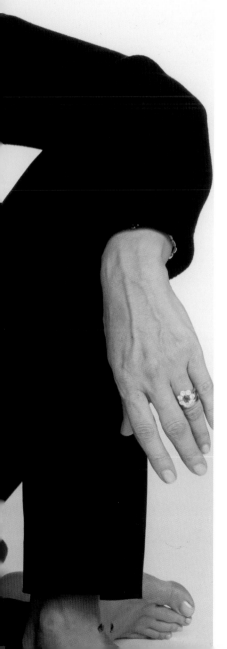

"I am never more beautiful than when I look into my children's faces."
—Lorraine Bracco

Lorraine Bracco with her daughters Margaux (left) and Stella.

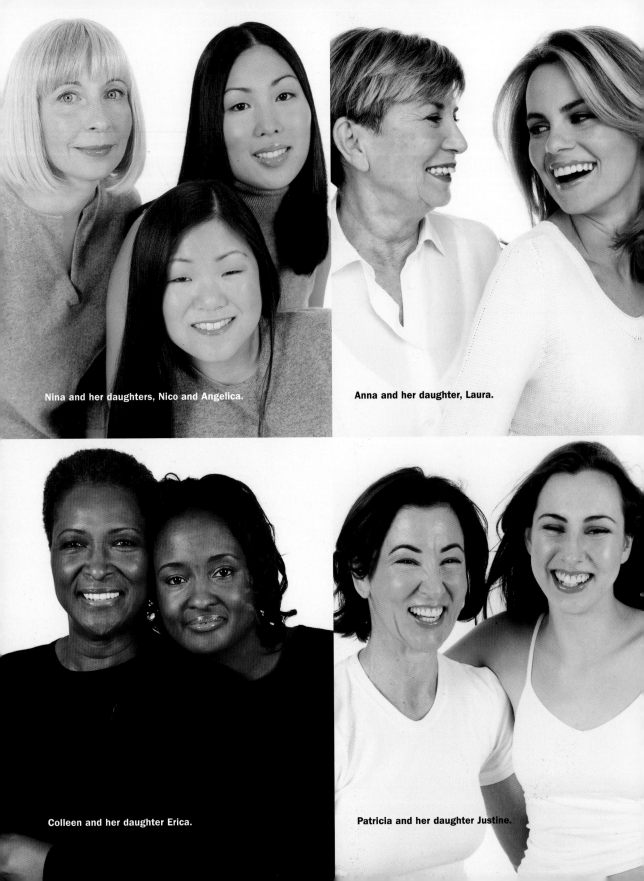

Nina and her daughters, Nico and Angelica.

Anna and her daughter, Laura.

Colleen and her daughter Erica.

Patricia and her daughter Justine.

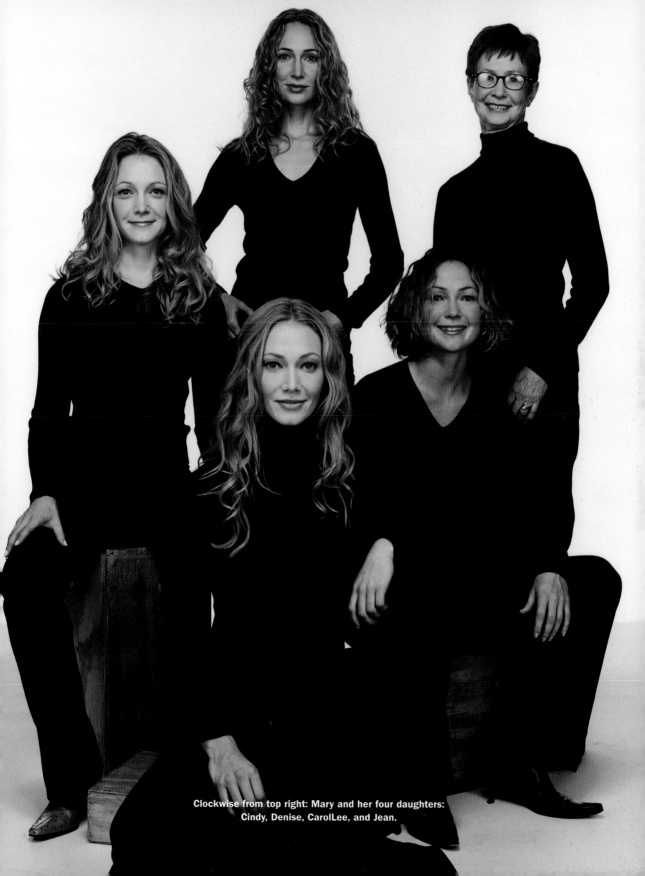

Clockwise from top right: Mary and her four daughters:
Cindy, Denise, CarolLee, and Jean.

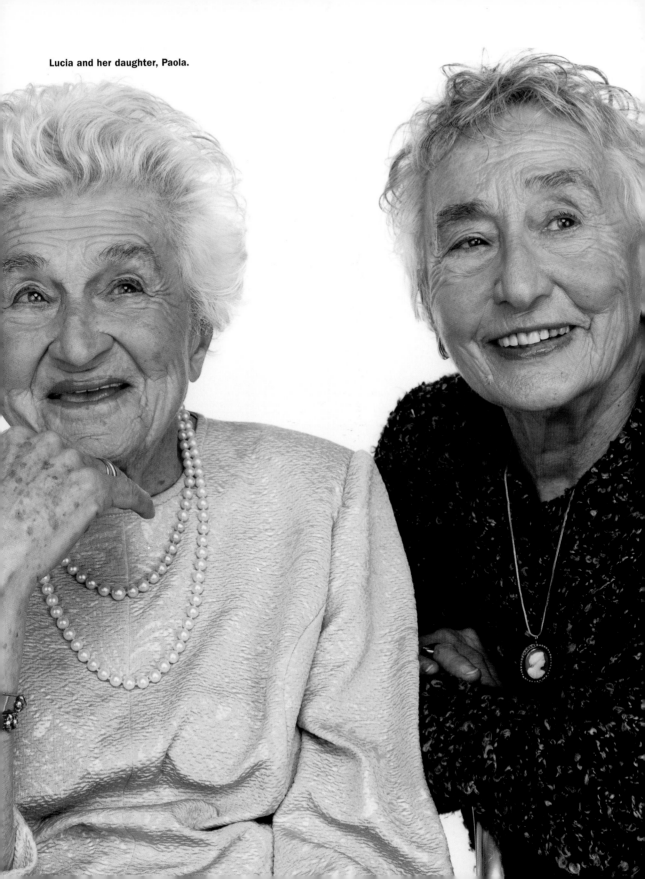

Lucia and her daughter, Paola.

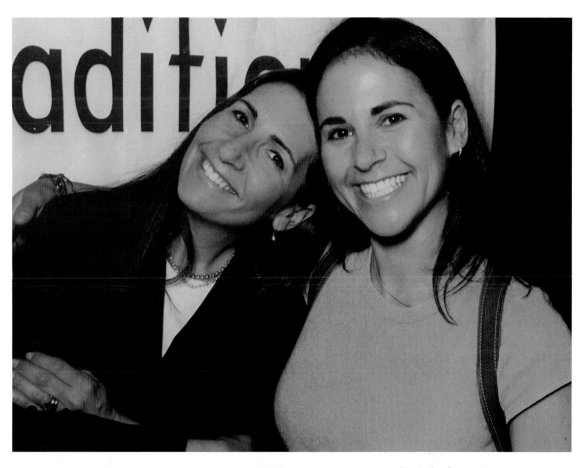

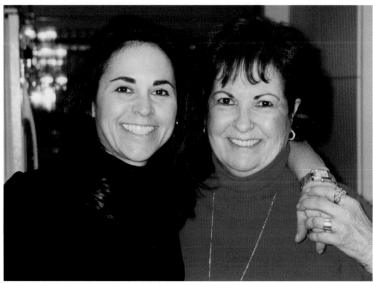

Clockwise from top:
me with my sister, Linda Arrandt;
me with our mom, Sandra Cain, and
Linda and Mom.

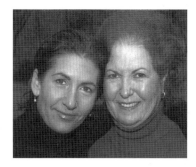

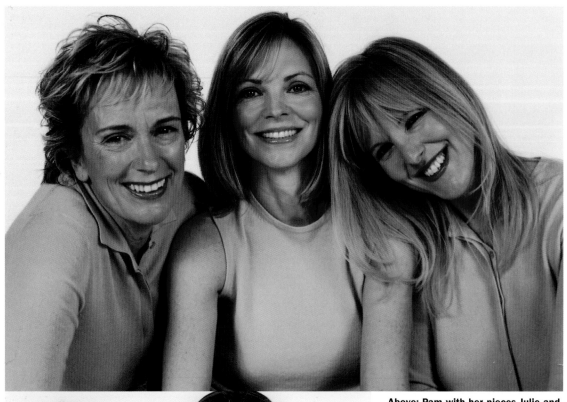

Above: Pam with her nieces Julie and Stacey.

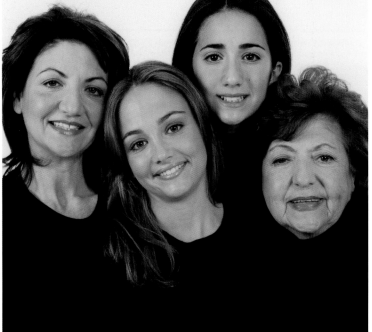

Left: Barbara with her daughters Tara and Nicole and her mother, Sylvia.

Right: The beautiful brother-and-sisters singing group, the Corrs.

206

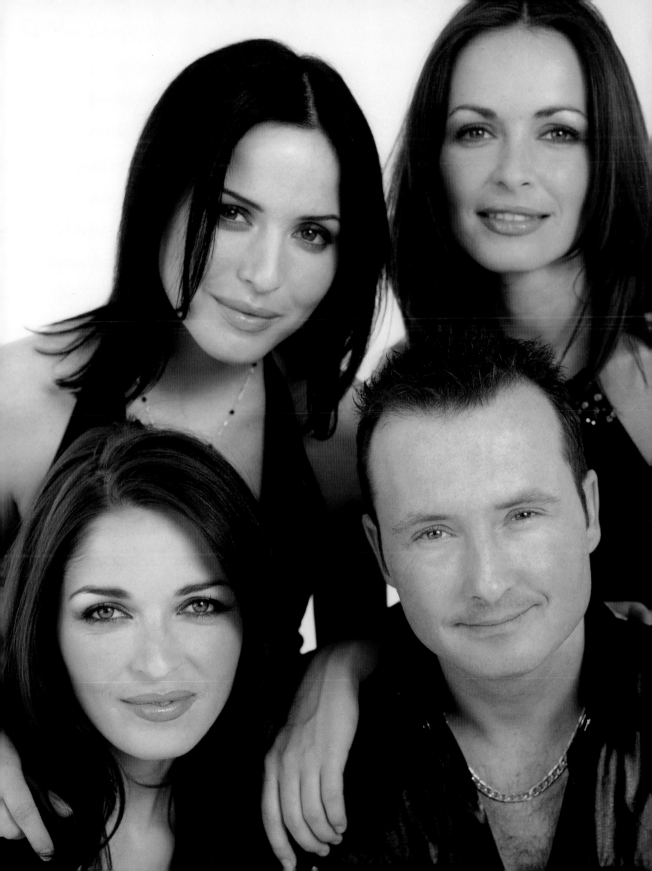

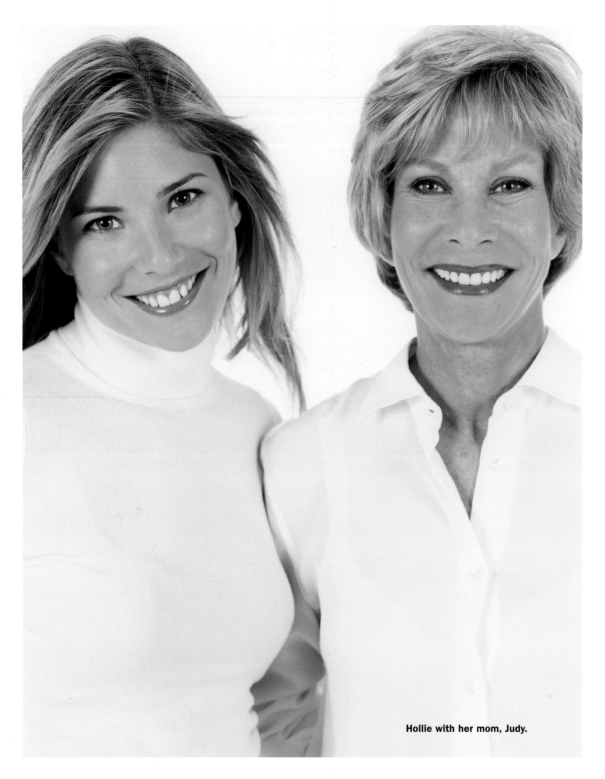

Hollie with her mom, Judy.

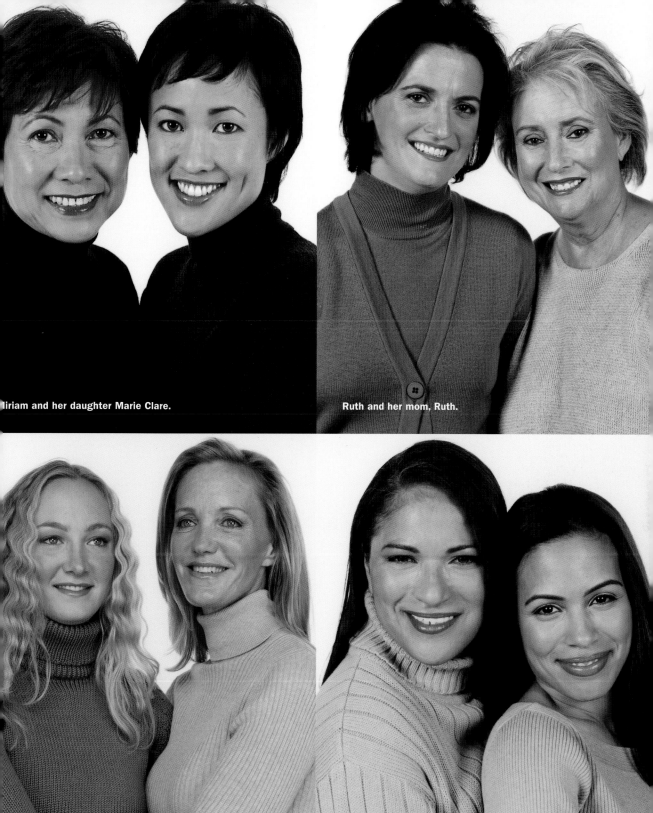

Miriam and her daughter Marie Clare.

Ruth and her mom, Ruth.

Emily and her mom, Martha.

Sandra and her daughter, Angie.

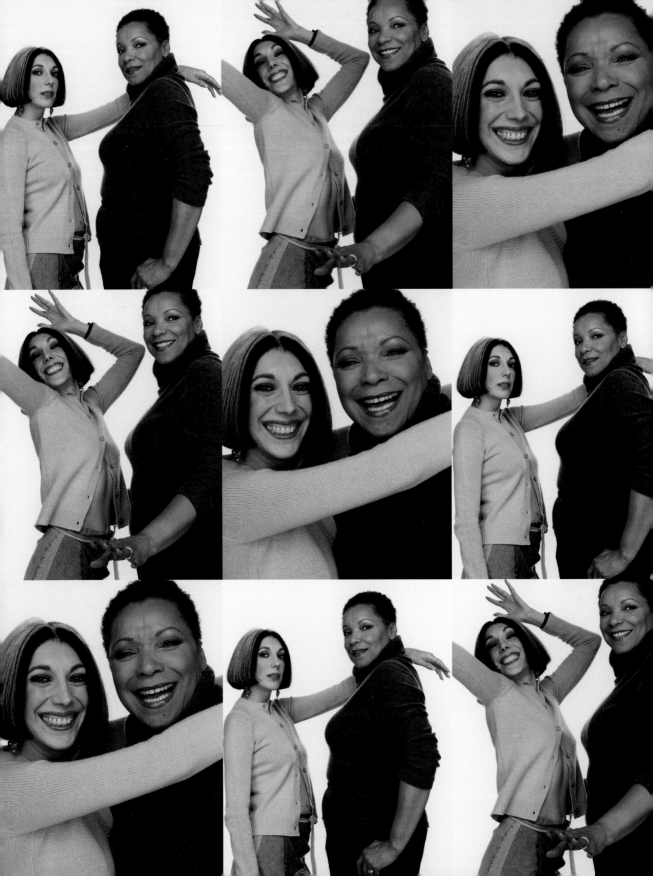

32 BEAUTY IS A LIFELONG EVOLUTION

I think it's natural to look at our flaws, but I'd like to think that it's possible to shift our focus toward looking at what's right with ourselves. (Just think how much happier you'd be as you face the mirror every morning.) If there is one overall message I want everyone to take away from this book, it is appreciate yourself now! Don't think about how good you used to look or how much better your life might be at some distant date in the future. For example, when I was in high school, I hated my arms. Now I look back at pictures of the past twenty years and think that my arms looked fine. Why was I avoiding sleeveless shirts? And probably in twenty more years, I'll look back and think the same about myself now. But why should we waste so much time and energy wishing for what used to be or might be later on? Your life, your looks, the good and the bad experiences are constantly evolving. And it's all good—provided you maintain the right attitude. That's why I chose so many real women of all ages to model for this book. The aim was to show how incredibly beautiful every stage of life can be. I hope you found these women as inspirational as I did.

Of course, anyone can look better. And hopefully, you've just learned a lot of the tricks I picked up over the years and put into these pages. But the bottom line is, beauty and makeup are not the most important things in the world. Take a deep breath, relax, and smile. I guarantee you look better already!

If there is one overall message I want everyone to take away from this book, it is appreciate yourself now!

photograph credits

Bobbi Brown's personal collection: v, ix, 2 (all), 3 (all), 4, 5 (left and right), 197 (bottom right), 205 (all). **Mark Babushkin:** 5 (middle). **Rick Burda:** 73, 74 (top), 84, 86 (all), 87 (all), 88, 89, 90, 92, 96, 100, 102, 103 (left), 110, 121, 170. **Rose Cali's personal collection:** 53 (top). **Walter Chin:** 6, 7, 10, 14, 18, 19, 22, 24 (bottom left, top right, and bottom right), 26, 28 (all), 29, 30, 31, 32, 34, 35 (top left, top right, and bottom left), 36 (all), 37 (all), 38, 41 (top left, bottom left, and bottom right), 42, 43, 44, 47 (top left and bottom right), 48 (both), 49 (all), 50, 58, 60 (both), 61, 62, 64, 65, 66, 70, 74 (bottom), 75, 76, 79, 81, 99, 101 (top), 104, 107, 109, 112 (right), 116, 117 (both), 118, 119, 120, 123 (both), 126, 128, 132 (bottom), 133, 134 (bottom left), 136, 137 (both), 138, 140 (both), 141 (middle and bottom), 143, 144 (all), 145, 148 (top left and right), 151 (bottom left and right), 153, 154, 155, 156 (bottom), 157 (top), 159, 160 (all), 165, 176, 192, 194 (top right and bottom left), 197 (top left), 198, 200-201, 202 (top right), 203, 204, 209 (bottom left), 210 (all). **Bernice Feldman and Selma Rosen's personal collection:** 11, 12, 13 (all). **Todd France:** 207. **G.K. & Vikki Hart/PhotoDisc/Getty Images:** 166. **Judy Kaufman's personal collection:** 173 (both). **Joe Pugliese:** 63. **Trudy Schlecter:** 197 (top right). **Ernesto Urdaneta:** x, 17 (bottom left), 23, 98 (both), 101 (bottom), 103 (right), 105, 106 (all), 108, 112 (left), 113 (all), 114, 115, 122 (bottom), 134 (top right), 146 (both), 147, 148 (bottom left and right), 151 (top left and right), 156 (top). **Lise Varrette:** xii, 16 (all), 17 (top left, top right, and bottom right), 20, 24 (middle right), 25, 35 (bottom right), 41 (top right), 46, 47 (top right and bottom left), 52, 53 (bottom), 54 (both), 55 (all), 56 (all), 57, 124, 125, 127, 130, 131, 135, 141 (top), 149 (all), 150 (all), 175, 179, 181, 182, 184 (all), 186 (both), 188 (both), 189 (all), 190, 191 (both), 194 (top left and bottom right), 202 (top left, bottom left, and bottom right), 206 (both), 208, 209 (top left, top right, and bottom right). **Carol Waksal:** 197 (bottom left). **Troy Word:** 8 (both), 9 (both), 122 (top and middle), 129 (all), 132 (top), 134 (bottom right), 152, 157 (middle and bottom), 158.